GLORIA L. BARR

When You Don't Sleep, Drink or Breathe

Historical, Shocking Short Stories Showing Why You Should Listen To Dr. Michael Breus

Copyright © 2024 by Gloria L. Barr

All rights reserved. No part of this publication may be reproduced, stored or transmitted in any form or by any means, electronic, mechanical, photocopying, recording, scanning, or otherwise without written permission from the publisher. It is illegal to copy this book, post it to a website, or distribute it by any other means without permission.

Printed in the United States of America

First edition

This book was professionally typeset on Reedsy.
Find out more at reedsy.com

Contents

1	The Exploits of Johann Goethe and His Fatal Breathing...	1
2	The Mysterious Insomnia of Emperor Wu of Han	7
3	The Unseen Cost of Queen Christina of Sweden's Extreme...	13
4	The Bizarre Case of the 'Mad' Artist Richard Dadd	19
5	The Sleeping Sickness that Doomed the Sultan of Zanzibar	25
6	The Mysterious Death of Princess Louise of Prussia:...	31
7	The Forgotten Case of the Italian Philosopher Who Starved to...	37
8	The Sleep Deprivation of Civil War Soldier Ambrose Bierce	43
9	The Breathing Collapse of John Keats	49
10	The Stress-Fueled Death of Alexander the Great	54
11	The Destructive Obsession of Captain Cook with Perfect...	60
12	The Tragic Downfall of the Earl of Essex Due to Sleep...	65
13	The Psychological Cost of the 1918 Spanish Flu on Public...	71
14	The Unseen Cost of Living Without Sleep in Ancient Egypt	77
15	The Final Days of Beethoven: Hydration and Overwork...	83

Contents

1. The Exploits of Johann Goethe and His Fatal Breathing... 1
2. The Mysterious Insomnia of Emperor Wu of Han 7
3. The Unseen Cost of Queen Christina of Sweden's Extreme... 13
4. The Bizarre Case of the 'Mad' Artist Richard Dadd 19
5. The Sleeping Sickness that Doomed the Sultan of Zanzibar 25
6. The Mysterious Death of Princess Louise of Prussia:... 31
7. The Forgotten Case of the Italian Philosopher Who Starved to... 37
8. The Sleep Deprivation of Civil War Soldier Ambrose Bierce 43
9. The Breathing Collapse of John Keats 49
10. The Stress-Fueled Death of Alexander the Great 54
11. The Destructive Obsession of Captain Cook with Perfect... 60
12. The Tragic Downfall of the Earl of Essex Due to Sleep... 65
13. The Psychological Cost of the 1918 Spanish Flu on Public... 71
14. The Unseen Cost of Living Without Sleep in Ancient Egypt 77
15. The Final Days of Beethoven: Hydration and Overwork... 83

1

The Exploits of Johann Goethe and His Fatal Breathing Experiment

Johann Wolfgang von Goethe, the towering figure of German literature and philosophy, is perhaps best known for his monumental works such as Faust and The Sorrows of Young Werther.

His intellectual legacy spans across poetry, drama, science, and the arts, influencing countless thinkers and artists for generations. But Goethe's eccentricities extended far beyond his literary genius—his fascination with the human body and mind led him down a path of self-experimentation that would border on the reckless and, at times, perilous. One of the most bizarre chapters of Goethe's life involved his exploration of breathing techniques, an experiment that would nearly cost him his life and raise questions about the balance between intellectual curiosity and personal safety.

The Quest for Clarity and Creativity

Goethe's interest in the mind-body connection was not just academic; it was deeply personal. Throughout his life, Goethe pursued a range of intellectual and physical activities, from studying anatomy to experimenting with color theory. But one of his most unusual fascinations lay in the power of breath—specifically, how control over one's breathing could potentially enhance creativity, clarity of thought, and even health.

Goethe believed that the human capacity for self-awareness was closely tied to the breath. He was particularly influenced by the idea that the breath, as a life force, could shape mental and emotional states. This belief was not unique to Goethe; throughout history, various cultures and spiritual traditions have seen breathing as a gateway to greater understanding. Yet Goethe's approach was not rooted in any religious or philosophical doctrine. Instead, it was grounded in his own experimentation, blending scientific inquiry with the kind of personal insight only a man of his intellectual stature could muster.

The Carbon Dioxide Experiment

In the late 18th and early 19th centuries, the science of respiration was still in its infancy. Scientists were only beginning to understand the role of gases like oxygen and carbon dioxide in the body's metabolic processes. Goethe, ever the curious mind, sought to apply this new knowledge to his own life. His most famous experiment involved intentionally limiting his intake of oxygen and increasing his exposure to carbon dioxide in an attempt to reach a heightened state of mental clarity.

The experiment was simple in theory but dangerous in practice. Goethe would place himself in small, enclosed spaces and deliberately alter his breathing patterns. He would reduce the volume of air he inhaled, attempting to create a feeling of euphoria and mental sharpness. At one point, he even confined himself to a closed room, exhaling the air and allowing the carbon dioxide to accumulate around him in a misguided attempt to improve his creativity.

Goethe's writings from this period, including his *Autobiography*, reflect his enthusiasm for the experiment. He described the process as an intense yet thrilling journey, one in which he sought to transcend the ordinary limitations of the human body and unlock a greater realm of mental potential. He wrote: "Through the control of the breath, I seek to regulate the flow of my thoughts, to silence the distractions of the world and reach a state of pure clarity."

However, Goethe's increasingly risky approach came with a dark consequence. As he pushed the boundaries of his experiment, his health began to deteriorate. The deliberate exposure to carbon dioxide—essentially depriving his body of oxygen for prolonged periods—left him weak, dizzy, and at times, nearly unconscious. His once robust physical health began to suffer, and the very creativity he sought to unlock became clouded by the ill effects of his self-imposed experiment.

Concern from Friends and Colleagues

Goethe's closest friends and colleagues, including the poet Friedrich Schiller, became alarmed by his behavior. Schiller, who had always admired Goethe's intellectual prowess, began to express concern as he noticed the toll the experiments were taking on his friend's physical and mental well-being. Schiller wrote in a letter to a mutual acquaintance: "Goethe has become consumed by his quest for enlightenment through breath, but I fear that it may lead him down a path from which he may not return."

Schiller, along with other contemporaries, urged Goethe to abandon his experiment. They pointed out the obvious dangers of his methods, including the risk of suffocation, and warned him that no amount of creative insight could justify endangering his life. Yet, Goethe was undeterred, convinced that he was on the cusp of an intellectual breakthrough.

The public, too, was both fascinated and disturbed by Goethe's eccentricities. At the time, Goethe was already a figure of immense cultural importance, and any action he took was closely scrutinized by the press. Newspapers reported on his self-experimentation with a mixture of awe and disbelief. One journalist wrote: "Goethe, in his relentless pursuit of perfection, has become a living experiment in the power of the mind over the body. But can the mind truly conquer the body, or is it a fool's errand?"

While some viewed Goethe's experiment as an inspiring act of intellectual courage, others saw it as reckless, a reflection of the very hubris that often accompanies genius. Public opinion on his activities was divided, with some hailing him as a visionary and others warning that his obsession with the limits of the human body could lead to disaster.

The Physical and Mental Toll

As Goethe continued his dangerous experiment, his health continued to decline. His once-sharp mind became clouded by dizziness and bouts of weakness. He experienced difficulty concentrating, and his ability to write with the same clarity and brilliance as before diminished. His physical appearance also suffered. Those who saw him during this period remarked on his pallor and the hollow look in his eyes, as though he were slowly withdrawing from the physical world in pursuit of an intellectual ideal.

At one point, Goethe's self-experimentation took a near-fatal turn. After an extended period of exposure to carbon dioxide, he became faint and nearly lost consciousness. His body had been deprived of oxygen for so long that his vital functions were beginning to shut down. Fortunately, Goethe was able to stop the experiment before it claimed his life, but the experience left him shaken and forced him to confront the dangers of his methods.

Despite the warnings from friends and the deterioration of his health, Goethe remained adamant about his belief that the breath was a key to unlocking higher states of creativity and consciousness. However, the risks he took in his personal experiments would later be seen as not only reckless but potentially fatal.

Modern Science and Understanding

Today, Goethe's experiment would be viewed through the lens of modern physiology and psychology. Carbon dioxide exposure is known to have significant effects on the human body, including dizziness, confusion, and, in extreme cases, loss of consciousness or death. Breathing exercises, though widely accepted for their calming and health benefits, are now understood to work best when practiced with awareness and balance—something Goethe's methods, rooted in intellectual fervor, lacked.

In the modern era, doctors and psychologists would likely have advised Goethe to seek more controlled and scientifically sound methods of exploring mental clarity. Methods such as controlled breathing, meditation, and mindfulness have been shown to have benefits without the associated risks of self-induced hypoxia. The idea of using breath to influence thought is still relevant today, but with an understanding of the body's limits and the necessity of maintaining a balanced approach.

Goethe's Legacy and the Costs of Eccentricity

Johann Wolfgang von Goethe ultimately abandoned his risky breathing experiments, but the legacy of his eccentricities endures. His relentless pursuit of intellectual and personal growth, though at times dangerous, serves as a testament to the intensity with which he approached life and thought. Today, Goethe's life is celebrated not only for his artistic and literary achievements but also for the unflinching nature of his intellectual curiosity. His experiments with breath may have been misguided, but they reflect the same drive that led to his greatest works.

2

The Mysterious Insomnia of Emperor Wu of Han

```
Emperor Wu of Han, one of the most powerful and influential
figures in Chinese history, ruled from 141 to 87 BCE.
```

His reign is often remembered for its military conquests, territorial expansion, and the establishment of the imperial bureaucracy. However, beneath his illustrious political achievements, Emperor Wu faced a hidden, debilitating struggle: chronic insomnia. This seemingly mundane health issue would not only plague the Emperor for decades but also have a profound effect on his rule and the stability of the Han dynasty. His inability to sleep spiraled into a medical crisis that undermined his decision-making, caused erratic governance, and contributed to his eventual downfall.

A Kingdom Built on Sleeplessness

The story of Emperor Wu's insomnia begins not with a single sleepless night, but with a prolonged and progressive disturbance to his sleep. Records of the Grand Historian by Sima Qian, one of the most valuable sources of historical information on the Han dynasty, suggests that Emperor Wu began to suffer from sleep deprivation during the later years of his reign. By the time he had consolidated his power and embarked on his ambitious military campaigns, his inability to sleep had become a serious issue.

Despite the many accomplishments of Emperor Wu, his health became increasingly fragile. The insomnia reportedly started when he was in his mid-thirties, soon after the tumultuous consolidation of power during his early reign. His life, filled with constant warfare, political strife, and personal anxiety, took a toll on his physical and mental state. According to Sima Qian's accounts, Emperor Wu found it increasingly difficult to achieve restful sleep, and his nights were often filled with restlessness, nightmares, and periods of complete wakefulness. At the time, medical understanding of sleep disorders was rudimentary at best, and the emperor's refusal to address the issue seriously only exacerbated the problem.

The Impact of Insomnia on His Mental Health

Sleep deprivation can severely affect cognitive function, and for Emperor Wu, the consequences were far-reaching. Insomnia led to heightened paranoia and increasing difficulty in distinguishing between reality and his delusions. Court physicians, notably Zhang Zhongjing, a renowned doctor of the time, repeatedly tried to intervene, offering various herbal remedies and calming teas. But Emperor Wu, driven by the urgency of his rule, would not rest. He believed his sleepless nights were a necessary sacrifice for the greatness of the empire.

Over time, his mental state deteriorated. Historical records describe the emperor as becoming suspicious of those around him, including his closest advisors and family members. His paranoia grew so intense that he began to distrust his own generals and military leaders, even accusing them of treachery without evidence. One famous incident involved his distrust of General Wei Qing, who had been instrumental in securing victories in the Xiongnu campaigns. Emperor Wu's insomnia caused him to view Wei Qing's successes with increasing suspicion, leading to a bitter conflict between the two that nearly resulted in Wei Qing's downfall.

His sleeplessness also led to emotional instability. On one occasion, it is reported that the Emperor had an outburst of anger against his ministers, accusing them of treachery, only to apologize moments later for his outburst, blaming it on his "restless nights." This emotional volatility undermined his authority, leaving his court unsettled and his advisors hesitant to voice dissent. Emperor Wu's once-clear decision-making became muddled by his lack of sleep, and his judgment became erratic.

Court Physicians and the Emperor's Refusal to Rest

Throughout the reign of Emperor Wu, court physicians and scholars attempted to address his insomnia with various remedies. They recommended dietary changes, herbal concoctions, and even acupuncture treatments to restore his sleep. One of the most famous figures in Han medicine, Zhang Zhongjing, was summoned to the emperor's court and prescribed a variety of treatments. Yet, despite these efforts, Emperor Wu resisted. His intense commitment to his work and the empire's demands, combined with his own obsession with immortality, led him to neglect his health.

At one point, Emperor Wu consulted with the famous Taoist sage and alchemist, Xu Hong, who was known for his expertise in elixirs of immortality. Xu Hong presented the emperor with a series of potions designed to restore his vitality and grant him eternal life. While these elixirs had no genuine medicinal value, their role in Emperor Wu's mental decline cannot be overstated. The obsession with finding a cure for his insomnia through mystical means only deepened his paranoia and irrationality.

Xu Hong's advice, though grounded in the mystical traditions of Taoism, was embraced by the emperor, who had begun to believe that the key to his eternal reign lay in his ability to conquer his physical limitations. His belief in these magical remedies further distorted his perception of reality, and his once-rational decisions became increasingly erratic.

The Political Fallout of Sleep Deprivation

Emperor Wu's insomnia took a tangible toll on his governance. His sleep-deprived mind often led him to make decisions without properly weighing the consequences. A notable example of this is his handling of the Xiongnu crisis. The Xiongnu, a powerful nomadic tribe to the north, posed a serious threat to the stability of the Han Empire. Emperor Wu, seeking to expand his territory and secure the empire's borders, initiated a series of military campaigns that stretched the empire's resources thin.

At the time, the Xiongnu were formidable foes, and their raids had a devastating impact on the northern regions of the empire. While military leaders like General Wei Qing were advocating for strategic restraint and negotiation, Emperor Wu's sleepless nights led him to push for increasingly aggressive tactics. His obsession with conquest, perhaps exacerbated by his inability to rest, led to campaigns that drained the empire's coffers and exhausted its military.

It is said that his insomnia contributed to his hasty decisions, making it difficult for him to listen to counsel or consider alternative strategies. His reign, which began with such promise and success, became marked by overreach and desperation. Military losses mounted, and discontent spread among the populace, who began to feel the effects of Emperor Wu's erratic policies.

The Deteriorating Public Opinion

As the years went on, Emperor Wu's insomnia and mental deterioration became more apparent, even to the public. It wasn't just his ministers who noticed his increasingly irrational behavior; the common people also saw the shift. In times of peace, the emperor had been known for his efforts to improve the lives of the people, implementing agricultural reforms and promoting the arts. But under the influence of chronic insomnia, Emperor Wu grew distant from the needs of his subjects.

Reports from the time, though fragmentary, suggest that the emperor's paranoia led him to increasingly view the population as a potential threat. In a particularly troubling incident, he ordered the execution of several prominent scholars who had publicly criticized his recent policies. These executions, driven by his sleepless nights and increasing sense of paranoia, sent shockwaves throughout the empire. The Han dynasty, once a symbol of order and prosperity, began to show signs of instability.

Public opinion shifted from admiration to fear. People began to see Emperor Wu not as the brilliant leader who had expanded the empire but as a man slowly succumbing to the ravages of his own mind. His sleepless nights seemed to have stripped him of his once-clear vision for the future, and his reign, once hailed as a golden age, began to falter.

The End of an Era: How Insomnia Contributed to His Downfall

Emperor Wu's insomnia didn't just affect his leadership during his reign—it also played a significant role in his eventual downfall. By the time he reached his final years, his health was in steep decline. His insomnia had given way to physical ailments, and his once-commanding presence had been replaced by an anxious, erratic ruler who could no longer hold the empire together.

Sima Qian's *Records of the Grand Historian* paints a grim picture of Emperor Wu in his later years. Descriptions from those who served him during this time suggest that his insomnia left him physically frail, emotionally unstable, and increasingly paranoid. He had isolated himself from the court, often refusing to listen to his advisors or hear the concerns of his people. His once-clear decisions became clouded by his inability to rest, and his mind, which had once been sharp and strategic, had become worn down by decades of sleepless nights.

Emperor Wu passed away in 87 BCE, and his death marked the end of an era for the Han dynasty. The empire he had built was left in a precarious position, with political instability beginning to take root. His insomnia, a silent but ever-present force in his life, had ultimately contributed to his inability to govern effectively in his final years. Though his reign had been marked by impressive military victories and territorial expansion, his inability to sleep left an indelible mark on the history of the Han dynasty—a reminder of the profound effects that physical and mental health can have on the course of history.

3

The Unseen Cost of Queen Christina of Sweden's Extreme Fasting

Queen Christina of Sweden remains one of the most enigmatic and unconventional monarchs in European history.

Born in 1626, Christina ascended to the throne at the tender age of six and ruled with an eccentricity that both fascinated and appalled those around her. As queen, she championed the arts and sciences, welcomed renowned thinkers like René Descartes to her court, and was known for her refusal to marry and take a traditional role as a ruler. But beneath her many intellectual pursuits and unconventional lifestyle lay a struggle with her own body, one that would ultimately contribute to her premature abdication and health decline.

One of the most striking and little-discussed aspects of Queen Christina's life was her extreme fasting regimen. Her obsession with maintaining a slender figure and mental clarity led her to adopt an increasingly restrictive diet, often going without food or water for extended periods. While fasting was a practice that had been revered by some religious figures and philosophers, Christina's approach was extreme, even by the standards of her time.

This extreme fasting, combined with a disregard for proper nourishment, would have a profound effect on her health and wellbeing, contributing to the breakdown of her physical and mental state. The consequences of her extreme habits were not only visible in her deteriorating health but also in the way her contemporaries, including prominent figures like René Descartes, reacted with concern.

The Queen's Obsession with Body and Mind

Queen Christina's fasting habits did not begin as a conscious decision to harm herself, but as part of an obsession with maintaining mental clarity and physical perfection. As a monarch, Christina faced constant pressure to be the ideal figurehead of the Swedish state, a responsibility that she found both suffocating and constricting. She was highly aware of her image and appearance, and in an era where royal figures were expected to maintain a carefully curated public persona, Christina took extreme measures to control her physical form.

Letters from her contemporaries reveal a queen who was profoundly concerned with her weight and appearance. In the court of the Swedish monarchy, she was known to have frequently commented on the importance of maintaining a "perfect" figure. Her court physicians warned her that her extreme fasting would eventually lead to serious health problems, but Christina remained unfazed. She continued with increasingly severe fasts, sometimes eating only a small amount of food every few days, while also restricting her water intake for extended periods.

This obsession with fasting was not merely about her body, however. Queen Christina believed that restricting her intake of food and water would help her focus her mind and maintain the intellectual sharpness she valued above all else. A deeply intellectual person, she sought mental clarity above all else and looked to fasting as a way to heighten her thinking. She saw herself as above the common constraints of the body, focusing instead on philosophical and scholarly pursuits.

Her obsession with mental clarity was not unique to her era. The concept of fasting as a means of enhancing cognition was a widely debated topic during the 17th century. Renowned philosophers such as René Descartes and others in her court often discussed the relationship between the body and mind. Descartes, who had become a close advisor to Christina during her reign, would later express concern over the queen's physical decline, advising her to abandon her extreme fasting habits. Despite his advice, Christina remained committed to her unusual lifestyle, believing that it was a necessary part of her intellectual journey.

René Descartes and the Queen's Decline

René Descartes, the famous French philosopher and mathematician, became one of Christina's closest confidants and advisors after she invited him to her court in 1649. Christina, ever the inquisitive mind, was drawn to Descartes' ideas on rationalism and the relationship between the body and the mind. She hoped that his intellectual guidance could help her understand the world in a new way, but over time, Descartes would become increasingly alarmed by her deteriorating health.

In letters to his colleagues, Descartes voiced his concern about Christina's health, particularly her extreme fasting. He expressed that he had warned her against such practices, explaining that they were dangerous and could lead to long-term health complications. Descartes even suggested that she was not only endangering her physical health but also jeopardizing her intellectual abilities. However, Christina dismissed his warnings and continued her extreme lifestyle, convinced that she could somehow transcend the physical limitations of her body.

It is believed that Descartes became so concerned about her condition that he urged the Swedish court to intervene. Despite his efforts, Christina's health continued to decline, and her extreme fasting became a source of tension between her and her advisors. Descartes, who had come to admire Christina for her intellect and her free-spirited approach to life, grew increasingly frustrated by her refusal to heed his advice.

His disillusionment with the queen was profound, and he began to distance himself from her, eventually leaving the Swedish court in 1650. Sadly, Descartes would die shortly after his departure from Sweden, but his concerns about Christina's health remained a point of contention in the court.

Public Reaction to Christina's Extreme Practices

Queen Christina's unorthodox lifestyle and fasting practices did not go unnoticed by the Swedish public. Her refusal to marry, her focus on intellectual pursuits, and her extreme dietary habits drew the attention of both critics and admirers. While some praised her for breaking traditional gender roles and focusing on intellectual pursuits, others viewed her as eccentric and out of touch with the realities of life as a monarch.

Swedish nobility and members of the court were often shocked by Christina's refusal to conform to the expectations of royal life. For example, her constant fasting made her seem increasingly frail and aloof, and her failure to produce an heir became a source of gossip and criticism. Her refusal to marry was seen as a deliberate rejection of her royal duty, and many believed that her failure to conform to the traditional role of a queen—both in terms of her physical appearance and her behavior—damaged her credibility as a ruler.

There were even whispers that Christina's fasting was a form of rebellion against the expectations placed on her as a woman and a monarch. She sought to assert her power not only in the political sphere but also in her personal life, refusing to submit to the pressures of traditional femininity. Her extreme fasting became emblematic of her struggle to assert her intellectual and personal autonomy, but it also made her appear increasingly disconnected from the world around her.

By the time Christina began to show signs of physical deterioration, the public opinion about her health was divided. While some of her followers and intellectual admirers continued to support her, many members of the Swedish court began to grow increasingly critical. Rumors of her declining health spread quickly, and the public began to question whether her unorthodox lifestyle was, in fact, harming her.

As Christina's condition worsened, her ability to govern effectively became increasingly compromised. Her extreme fasting had made her more vulnerable to illness, and her advisors began to fear that her physical frailty would weaken her authority and, by extension, the stability of the monarchy. Despite her intellectual brilliance, Christina's ability to rule and make decisions was increasingly undermined by her physical and mental state.

The Abdication and Aftermath

In 1654, at the age of 28, Queen Christina made the unprecedented decision to abdicate the Swedish throne in favor of her cousin, Charles X Gustav. Her decision was widely regarded as a shock, as Christina had ruled Sweden for over two decades and was one of the most powerful monarchs in Europe at the time. While her abdication has been attributed to a variety of factors, including her disinterest in marriage and the burdens of rulership, it is likely that her declining health played a significant role in her decision.

By the time of her abdication, Christina's extreme fasting and refusal to properly nourish her body had taken a visible toll on her health. She had become increasingly frail and was unable to carry out her royal duties. Her abdication marked the end of an era for Sweden and, in many ways, the culmination of her struggle against the expectations of her role as a monarch.

After her abdication, Christina moved to Rome, where she continued to be an intellectual force, hosting salons and engaging with some of the greatest minds of her time. However, her health continued to deteriorate, and she passed away in 1689 at the age of 62—an early death for a queen who had once been at the height of her power. While Christina's intellectual legacy lived on, her extreme fasting practices and refusal to adhere to the basic needs of her body left an indelible mark on her life and reign. Her untimely death was, in many ways, a tragic reminder of the hidden costs of a life lived in extreme pursuit of both intellectual clarity and physical perfection.

4

The Bizarre Case of the 'Mad' Artist Richard Dadd

Richard Dadd, once considered one of the brightest artistic talents of Victorian England, is now remembered not just for his vivid and haunting paintings, but also for the tragic and bizarre events that led to his downfall.

His story is one that blurs the lines between genius and madness, a tale of how the intense pressures of artistic ambition, combined with sleep deprivation and substance abuse, spiraled into a violent act that shocked society. The murder of his father by Dadd, and his subsequent descent into insanity, remains one of the most disturbing chapters in the history of British art.

A Prodigy in the Making

Born in 1817, Richard Dadd was recognized early on as a gifted artist. His work was filled with intricate detail and vibrant scenes, and by his twenties, he had already gained attention for his remarkable skill. He became a prominent member of the Royal Academy, where his peers and professors admired his mastery of landscapes, portraits, and mythology. But beneath his outward success, Dadd was hiding a growing instability.

His fame as an artist took a sharp turn in the mid-1840s when he embarked on a journey to the Middle East. It was in Egypt, during this period, that his mental health began to deteriorate. The stress of travel, the extreme climate, and the demands of his work weighed heavily on him. More significantly, Dadd's growing obsession with mysticism and the supernatural began to consume him, setting the stage for his tragic fall.

The Hallucinations and the Breaking Point

Dadd's mental decline is often attributed to a combination of factors, most notably the extreme work schedule he kept during his early years. Dadd was known for his obsessive dedication to his craft, spending long hours, sometimes days, without rest, in pursuit of perfection. Sleep deprivation was a constant in his life, and during this time, he began to experience vivid hallucinations. His paintings, once rich in classical and serene landscapes, began to morph into strange, distorted worlds—visions of creatures from myth and folklore, and figures suspended between dream and reality.

The influence of drugs also cannot be underestimated in Dadd's downward spiral. The use of opium and other substances was common in the Victorian era, particularly among artists seeking inspiration or relief from stress. It is believed that Dadd's use of opium to ease the exhaustion brought on by sleep deprivation and his intense work schedule contributed to his deteriorating mental state. His already fragile grip on reality was loosened further by his increasing reliance on these substances, which in turn amplified his hallucinations.

By the time he returned to London in 1843, Dadd's delusions had become more intense and bizarre. He believed that he was the agent of God's will, tasked with eradicating evil from the world. His paranoia intensified, and he became fixated on the idea that his father, a well-regarded middle-class man, was a demonic figure. His father's attempts to intervene and stop his erratic behavior only worsened the situation.

The Murder of His Father

On August 28, 1843, Richard Dadd's mental state reached a tragic breaking point. In a delusional frenzy, he brutally murdered his father, stabbing him repeatedly in what he later described as an act of divine intervention. Dadd believed that by killing his father, he was fulfilling a divine command to rid the world of evil. In his fractured mind, the death was necessary, part of a larger cosmic battle.

After the murder, Dadd fled London, embarking on a journey to France and then to Belgium, where he was eventually apprehended. His crime quickly became a sensation in the press, with newspapers like *The Times* speculating on the causes of his breakdown. The murder of a prominent family member by a respected artist shocked the Victorian public, but what followed was perhaps even more disturbing. The press, fascinated by the murder and its grisly details, turned their attention to Dadd's psychological condition.

Many newspapers of the time were quick to sensationalize the event, with some speculating that Dadd had been driven mad by his work schedule, while others pointed to his increasing obsession with mystical beliefs and drug use. In a time when mental illness was often poorly understood, these sensational accounts did little to shed light on the true nature of his condition.

The Examination of Richard Dadd

When Dadd was eventually caught and brought to trial, the question of his sanity became central to the case. Victorian society, still grappling with the emerging field of psychology, was ill-equipped to understand the complexities of mental illness. Richard Dadd's case was one of the first to bring attention to the link between creative genius, sleep deprivation, and mental instability.

The physician who first examined Dadd was Dr. Thomas S. Clouston, a prominent figure in the history of psychiatry, who later became known for his studies of mental disorders. Clouston's report on Dadd's condition described a man suffering from acute paranoid delusions, whose mental state had been worsened by sleep deprivation, drug abuse, and stress. According to Clouston, Dadd's case was a clear example of how chronic exhaustion and substance abuse could unravel a person's mind.

Clouston was not alone in his assessment. Other doctors who treated Dadd at the time, including those at Bethlem Royal Hospital (also known as Bedlam), were equally concerned with the role of sleep deprivation in his breakdown. Dadd's lack of sleep, combined with his obsessive work habits and increasing paranoia, were seen as the key factors in his transformation from a promising artist into a man consumed by madness.

The Artistic Legacy of Richard Dadd

Despite the horrors of his crime and his prolonged confinement in the asylum, Richard Dadd continued to paint throughout his life. His works, produced while in prison, are often seen as a reflection of his fractured mind. His most famous piece, *The Fairy Feller's Master-Stroke*, is a detailed and bizarre representation of fairies and mythical creatures, executed with painstaking precision. The painting, now housed in the Tate Britain, is an eerie testament to the artist's unique vision, but also a chilling glimpse into the mind of a man who was no longer fully grounded in reality.

Many of Dadd's paintings, like *The Fairy Feller's Master-Stroke*, display an obsessive attention to detail, with characters and scenes that appear to be suspended between worlds. The intensity of his work, combined with the strangeness of the imagery, invites speculation about the artist's inner turmoil. Scholars and art historians have long debated whether Dadd's paintings reflect a brilliant mind unraveling or a deeper, more profound understanding of a reality beyond human comprehension.

While his paintings were celebrated for their technical mastery, they were also a reminder of the toll that his mental illness had taken on him. Today, Dadd is remembered as both a tragic figure and a remarkable artist whose life and work continue to provoke intrigue and discussion. His case serves as an example of the complex relationship between creativity and mental illness, highlighting the ways in which sleep deprivation and substance abuse can destroy not only a person's health but also their ability to function in the world.

Modern Psychological Understanding

Modern psychology offers a more nuanced understanding of Richard Dadd's condition, though the full complexity of his case remains a subject of debate. Today, it is understood that sleep deprivation, especially when chronic, can have profound effects on mental health. The symptoms of paranoia, hallucinations, and delusions that Dadd experienced are now known to be associated with conditions like schizophrenia and other psychotic disorders. Moreover, substance abuse, particularly the use of opiates, can exacerbate these symptoms, leading to an even greater breakdown of reality.

Dadd's case is a stark reminder of how fragile the mind can be, especially when subjected to extreme stress and exhaustion. In an era where mental illness was not well understood, his descent into madness was both a personal tragedy and a societal warning. Today, artists and creatives are often encouraged to maintain a balance between their work and their well-being, but for Richard Dadd, such guidance came too late. His legacy is one of brilliance shadowed by madness, a haunting reminder of the dangers of pushing oneself too far in the pursuit of artistic greatness.

5

The Sleeping Sickness that Doomed the Sultan of Zanzibar

In the late 19th century, the island of Zanzibar, an important trading hub off the east coast of Africa, found itself at the center of an unprecedented health crisis.

The epidemic that struck the region in the 1890s was one of the most bizarre and mysterious diseases of the time—an outbreak of *encephalitis lethargica*, commonly known as sleeping sickness. This rare and devastating illness, which caused widespread sleep deprivation, confusion, and in many cases, death, would have far-reaching consequences for the Sultanate of Zanzibar. The illness, coupled with the sultan's own deteriorating health, played a key role in the downfall of the sultan's dynasty, making this chapter of Zanzibar's history not only tragic but also deeply entwined with political and social instability.

A Mysterious Illness Strikes Zanzibar

The sleeping sickness that plagued Zanzibar in the late 1800s was a terrifying and puzzling epidemic. Symptoms of *encephalitis lethargica* included extreme drowsiness, confusion, fever, and the inability to stay awake for extended periods. Victims would enter long states of near-comatose sleep, often for days at a time, only to wake up disoriented and with significant cognitive impairment. In some cases, patients died while in their stupor, unable to fight off the infection. In others, the illness caused long-term neurological damage, leaving survivors with speech and movement disabilities.

The onset of the disease was sudden and brutal. People would fall ill with little warning, their lives turned upside down by the relentless effects of the illness. Families were torn apart, as they watched loved ones either slip into unconsciousness or endure severe mental disturbances. It was not just a disease of the body, but of the mind, and its victims were often left in a state of confusion and vulnerability that left them unable to care for themselves or their families.

At the time, no one understood the true cause of *encephalitis lethargica*. Some speculated that it was linked to an environmental factor, such as an outbreak of a particular toxin or a virulent strain of bacteria. Others saw it as a supernatural occurrence or divine punishment, particularly given the catastrophic impact the illness had on both the general population and the ruling class. For the people of Zanzibar, it was a cruel twist of fate that their suffering seemed to coincide with a period of great political upheaval.

THE SLEEPING SICKNESS THAT DOOMED THE SULTAN OF ZANZIBAR

The Sultan's Inability to Manage the Crisis

The Sultan of Zanzibar at the time of the epidemic was *Sultan Hamad bin Thuwaini*, who had ascended to the throne in 1870. Despite his attempts to maintain a semblance of control over his people, the outbreak of sleeping sickness caught him and his government unprepared. The Sultan, much like many of his European counterparts, lacked a clear understanding of the disease and was at a loss as to how to stop it.

The British, who had been exerting increasing influence over Zanzibar and the surrounding region, were deeply concerned by the spread of the illness. European powers were already wary of the region's instability and viewed the epidemic as a further sign that the Sultanate was teetering on the edge of collapse. British officials stationed in Zanzibar began to question whether the sultan was fit to govern, as the outbreak exposed the weak infrastructure and lack of resources in the Sultanate.

Newspapers such as *The Times* in London reported on the crisis, framing it as both a humanitarian tragedy and a political failure. Articles published during this period often painted a picture of a sultan who was struggling not only with the effects of the illness on his people but also with his own declining health. Sultan Hamad himself was not immune to the disease, and his health began to deteriorate in parallel with the spread of the epidemic. Reports from the time indicated that the Sultan, though weakened by illness, continued to carry out his duties, despite being visibly unwell. His inability to manage the crisis, both in terms of providing medical care and maintaining control over his government, further diminished his reputation.

The Public's View of the Sultan's Leadership

As the sleeping sickness spread throughout Zanzibar, public opinion of the Sultan began to sour. The people of Zanzibar, already living under the oppressive weight of colonial influence and political unrest, now found themselves facing the additional burden of a mysterious and deadly disease. Sultan Hamad's inability to stem the tide of illness was widely viewed as a failure of leadership, and his efforts to provide aid were seen as insufficient. The Sultan's reign, already marked by political fragility and increasing foreign influence, now faced a crisis that further exposed the weakness of his rule.

In the eyes of many, the Sultan was unable to protect his people from the illness, and his seeming indifference to their suffering eroded the support he had among his subjects. Local leaders and advisors, including members of his own court, began to question his competency, and rumors spread about his declining health. Sultan Hamad's physical decline mirrored the collapse of his authority, and the people's faith in his ability to govern waned.

European observers, particularly those from Britain, began to scrutinize the situation more closely. Their concern was not only for the wellbeing of the Sultan's subjects but for the potential political ramifications of a failed Sultanate. The colonial powers, especially Britain, had long sought to establish greater control over Zanzibar's strategic location, and the presence of a weak and incapacitated Sultan only heightened their sense of opportunity. British officials saw the Sultan's inability to manage the epidemic as a clear sign that his rule was ineffective and unable to handle crises of this scale.

The Sultan's Decline and the Collapse of the Dynasty

As the epidemic raged on, Sultan Hamad's health continued to deteriorate. Like many of his subjects, he succumbed to the physical and mental toll of the disease. While the illness claimed the lives of many of Zanzibar's inhabitants, it also marked the beginning of the end for Hamad's reign. The Sultan, who had once been regarded as a figure of strength and leadership, was now seen as weak and incapable of ruling.

The Sultan's physical collapse was followed by political instability. With the British keenly observing the unfolding crisis, they began to assert more control over Zanzibar. Sultan Hamad's decline left a power vacuum, and in 1893, just a few years after the peak of the epidemic, the Sultanate was formally placed under British protectorate status. Sultan Hamad's death in 1896 marked the end of his rule and the collapse of the Hamad dynasty. His successors, though still recognized as the nominal leaders of Zanzibar, would never regain the full power that the Sultanate had once held.

The spread of *encephalitis lethargica* had not only devastated the health of the people but had also undermined the political fabric of Zanzibar. The epidemic's arrival coincided with a period of growing colonial influence, and it served as a catalyst for the eventual annexation of Zanzibar by British authorities. The disease, though seemingly a natural disaster, became entwined with the politics of the time, serving as a grim metaphor for the declining fortunes of the Sultan's dynasty.

The Legacy of the Sleeping Sickness

The sleeping sickness epidemic in Zanzibar left behind a trail of tragedy, both in terms of human suffering and political upheaval. The disease, which caused untold pain and loss of life, played a significant role in the weakening of the Sultanate, hastening its decline and facilitating the expansion of colonial power in the region. The British, having long desired more control over Zanzibar, saw the epidemic as both a sign of the Sultanate's instability and an opportunity to further their interests.

Zanzibar's public opinion of Sultan Hamad's leadership, already fragile, plummeted during the epidemic. His inability to manage the crisis, combined with his own personal decline, sealed his fate as a ruler unable to protect his people. The outbreak of *encephalitis lethargica* not only claimed the lives of many but also marked the beginning of the end for the Hamad dynasty.

While the disease itself eventually faded, the legacy of the epidemic and the collapse of the Sultanate continued to reverberate in the political landscape of East Africa. The sleeping sickness that once seemed like a random affliction had, in many ways, sealed the fate of the Sultanate of Zanzibar, marking a turning point in the history of the region.

6

The Mysterious Death of Princess Louise of Prussia: Dehydration or Poison?

```
The sudden and unexplained death of Princess Louise of
Prussia in 1810 remains one of the most perplexing and
scandalous events in the annals of European royal history.
```

Princess Louise, daughter of King Friedrich Wilhelm II of Prussia, was a well-known figure in high society, famous for her beauty, wit, and extravagant lifestyle. However, her untimely demise, which occurred at the young age of 34, has been the subject of much speculation over the years. While some reports suggest her death was a result of extreme dehydration brought on by her neglect of personal health, others hinted at more sinister causes, including possible poisoning.

The circumstances surrounding Princess Louise's death have sparked heated debates among historians, medical experts, and conspiracy theorists alike. Was her demise truly the result of a failure to hydrate, or was it an insidious act of foul play? As rumors swirled throughout royal courts and across Europe, the tragic death of this beloved princess became an enigma that would take decades to even partially unravel.

A Life of Excess and Neglect

Princess Louise was a prominent figure in the royal courts of Europe, known not just for her noble heritage, but for her active participation in the social scene. She was a fixture of the lavish Prussian aristocracy, attending balls, dinner parties, and social gatherings. But her lifestyle was not without its consequences. Although she was admired for her beauty, intelligence, and charm, her personal habits were often seen as erratic and unhealthy. Most notably, her disregard for proper hydration was well known among her peers and physicians.

Despite the availability of water and the increasing understanding of health practices in the early 19th century, Princess Louise was often reported to neglect drinking enough fluids. Her royal physicians were concerned by her lack of interest in regular meals and liquids, with some noting that she frequently substituted water for alcohol or failed to drink altogether, particularly during social events when wine and champagne were more readily available.

Her disregard for hydration was not a solitary instance of poor self-care; Louise's overall lifestyle was one of indulgence. She was known to partake in late-night revelries and long days of social engagements, often at the expense of rest, healthy nutrition, and even basic hygiene. It was a lifestyle not uncommon among the European aristocracy, but it was one that would eventually take a toll on her health.

The Mysterious Illness

Princess Louise's health had been deteriorating for several months leading up to her sudden death. She had reportedly experienced bouts of extreme fatigue, headaches, and dizziness, but these symptoms were often dismissed as the result of stress or overwork. Royal physicians, familiar with her hectic schedule and indulgent lifestyle, did not initially express concern, believing her condition to be temporary. But as her symptoms grew worse, there was a distinct shift in diagnosis.

In the weeks before her death, Louise reportedly became more withdrawn and irritable. She often complained of nausea, stomach cramps, and dizziness, but insisted on continuing with her usual social engagements. One of the final reports from her personal doctor, Dr. Wilhelm von Goecking, mentioned that her lips had become dry and cracked, a clear sign of severe dehydration. But at the same time, the princess's deteriorating condition seemed to progress at an alarming rate, with her physical state worsening each day. She had lost significant weight and appeared visibly pale, a stark contrast to the vivacious woman who had once dominated social scenes across Europe.

On the morning of her death, Princess Louise collapsed in her private chambers. Doctors were quickly summoned, but they were too late. Louise had already slipped into a coma, and within hours, she was gone. Her sudden death sent shockwaves through the royal courts and beyond, leaving behind more questions than answers.

Theories of Poisoning and Public Speculation

At first, many believed Princess Louise's death was due to an unfortunate, but not entirely uncommon, illness. The rapidity of her decline, however, led to suspicions that something more sinister was at play. Among the rumors circulating throughout the courts, one of the most persistent was that Louise had been poisoned. This theory was not without precedent—poisoning had often been a tool used by ambitious rivals in royal circles.

Her sudden and dramatic decline in health, coupled with her strange symptoms, fueled these suspicions. While her symptoms—extreme fatigue, nausea, dizziness—could be explained by dehydration, they were also indicative of poisoning. Some in the court even pointed to the fact that Louise had been particularly sensitive to certain foods and drinks, raising the possibility that someone had laced her wine or food with toxins, such as arsenic or belladonna, which were commonly used in the 19th century.

Adding fuel to the fire, Princess Louise had a number of political and personal enemies, many of whom had reasons to see her out of the picture. Louise had been a significant political figure in her own right, and her close ties to the Prussian court had earned her the ire of some members of the nobility, particularly those who opposed the reforms and policies championed by her father, King Friedrich Wilhelm II.

However, the idea that her death was caused by poison was never definitively proven. In fact, royal physicians who examined her after her death found no evidence of foul play. The autopsy, which was carried out by Dr. Goecking and several other court doctors, revealed that Louise had been severely dehydrated. Her organs, particularly her kidneys and liver, showed signs of damage consistent with prolonged neglect of basic hydration.

Hydration or Poison: The Royal Debate

As the days passed after Princess Louise's death, the debate over whether her demise was due to dehydration or poison continued to grow. Newspapers in Europe began to publish speculative reports, some of which pointed to foul play. The *Berlin Gazette* reported that some members of the royal family were convinced that Louise's death had been the result of a political conspiracy, while others claimed she had succumbed to a long-standing illness.

The public, too, was divided. Some saw Louise's death as a tragic accident, the inevitable result of a life spent indulging in excess without proper regard for her health. Others believed her death was a consequence of the immense pressure placed on her by the royal family to conform to a rigid and demanding role that left little room for personal care. The very lifestyle that had once defined her image as a glamorous, charismatic princess had also contributed to her downfall.

Still, others whispered about the possibility of a darker explanation. The *Times of London* published an article questioning whether Louise's death was truly a result of dehydration, arguing that her social circle had become a "breeding ground for scandal" and that her sudden decline had too many unexplained elements. Were the symptoms of dehydration too convenient, they wondered, a perfect cover for a more calculated act of poisoning?

The Role of Hydration in the 19th Century

In the early 19th century, the medical understanding of hydration and its importance was still in its infancy. While doctors had begun to recognize the dangers of dehydration, the prevailing medical opinion of the time often underestimated its significance. Dehydration was frequently viewed as a secondary concern, overshadowed by more pressing health issues such as infectious diseases and fevers. Therefore, it is not entirely surprising that Princess Louise's physicians might have overlooked the importance of keeping her properly hydrated.

In a royal court where excess was the norm, it was far more common for the nobility to indulge in alcohol, rich food, and social distractions than in simple practices like drinking water. Louise's lifestyle, full of lavish banquets and constant socializing, made it easy for her to neglect her most basic needs. Her reliance on wine and champagne, combined with the absence of enough water, could easily have led to the kind of severe dehydration that contributed to her sudden collapse and death.

The Scandal and the Legacy

As the investigation into Princess Louise's death dragged on, the scandal surrounding her demise only deepened. Some claimed that the Prussian court had intentionally downplayed the role of dehydration in her death to avoid a public scandal, while others believed that the royal family itself had been too embarrassed to confront the possibility that a princess had died from something as preventable as dehydration.

In the years that followed, Louise's death was immortalized in the annals of royal history as a cautionary tale about the dangers of neglecting one's health in favor of excess. Her untimely passing raised important questions about the responsibilities of those in power to not only manage their political duties but to also care for their own well-being.

For some, Princess Louise's death symbolized the tragic consequences of a life lived in excess, and the inability to confront the realities of one's physical limitations. For others, it remained a mystery—a bizarre chapter in the storied history of European royalty, one that would never be fully solved.

7

The Forgotten Case of the Italian Philosopher Who Starved to Death

Giambattista Vico, the 18th-century philosopher from Naples, was an intellectual giant whose work laid the foundation for modern philosophy, history, and social theory.

H is ideas on the cyclical nature of history and his advocacy for the "new science" of understanding human civilization earned him recognition far beyond his time. However, the personal cost of his intellectual pursuits, particularly his obsession with writing, was tragically high. In his later years, Vico's relentless devotion to his work led to severe neglect of his physical health. His gradual descent into malnutrition and eventual starvation has long been a subject of sorrow among historians, intellectuals, and scholars.

Vico's case is a stark reminder of the dangers of intellectual obsession, showing how a brilliant mind can disregard the basic needs of the body in pursuit of ideas. The question remains: How could such a profound thinker neglect his own well-being so completely? What led Vico to abandon his health, and how did this affect his work and legacy?

An Obsession with Intellectual Work

Giambattista Vico was born in Naples in 1668, and by the early 18th century, he had already made a name for himself as a professor of rhetoric and a philosopher. However, it was his magnum opus, *Scienza Nuova* (The New Science), published in 1725, that would immortalize him in the intellectual canon. The book proposed a novel theory about the development of human civilization, emphasizing the cyclical nature of history and the importance of understanding culture through mythology, language, and societal structures.

While *The New Science* was groundbreaking, Vico's dedication to writing it—and his other intellectual pursuits—came at a great personal cost. He was notorious for his solitary, obsessive work habits. His passion for philosophy and history often consumed him completely, leading him to ignore physical discomfort, lack of sleep, and, most worryingly, his basic needs for food and water.

According to his contemporaries, Vico was rarely seen eating regular meals. His letters and personal accounts suggest that he would work for hours without pausing to eat, drinking only small amounts of water. He became known for working deep into the night, often foregoing dinner in favor of continuing to write and refine his theories. This lifestyle, typical of many 17th and 18th-century intellectuals who saw themselves as martyrs for the pursuit of knowledge, ultimately took a toll on his body.

The Decline of Health: A Slow Starvation

Vico's obsession with his work only intensified in the years after the publication of *Scienza Nuova*. As the philosopher grew older, his physical condition deteriorated. His excessive intellectual focus led to increasing physical neglect, and this neglect soon took the form of malnutrition. Though contemporary accounts differ, it is clear that Vico's lack of appetite, exacerbated by his tendency to forgo meals in favor of writing, had a significant impact on his health.

In one letter to a friend, Vico himself remarked that his physical condition had worsened, describing how he felt weak and listless yet unable to stop working. He referred to his body as a "ruined vessel," a reflection of his disregard for his health. Over time, this neglect manifested in more alarming ways: Vico became increasingly frail, his skin grew pale, and his mental clarity began to suffer. Even more concerning, his handwriting, once sharp and clear, became erratic, as if the strength to maintain such precision was beyond his grasp.

His friends and colleagues expressed growing concern. Among the most vocal was the Neapolitan physician and scholar Francesco D'Aguirre, who warned Vico that his refusal to maintain a healthy lifestyle would have catastrophic consequences. D'Aguirre wrote in a letter that he had tried on several occasions to persuade Vico to eat more regularly and to take better care of himself, but Vico remained stubbornly fixated on his work.

One of Vico's closest friends, the poet and philosopher Antonio Genovesi, also expressed deep concern. In a letter written in 1740, Genovesi remarked on how Vico's physical deterioration was "painfully evident," noting that his friend had lost considerable weight and was visibly exhausted. "His mind is still as sharp as ever," Genovesi wrote, "but his body is on the verge of collapse."

Despite these warnings, Vico continued to resist his friends' advice.

He was so deeply absorbed in his intellectual world that he failed to recognize the extent to which his body was breaking down. His devotion to his theories became a form of self-imposed martyrdom, where his philosophical mission was so vital to him that everything else—his health, his well-being, his life itself—was secondary.

The Public Reaction and Speculation

By the time Vico's health had deteriorated to its lowest point, public reaction was divided. For many, his intellectual contributions were too significant to be overshadowed by his personal decline. Some members of the intellectual community were quick to excuse his physical deterioration as the inevitable cost of genius. After all, figures like Descartes, Pascal, and others had similarly sacrificed their own physical comfort for the sake of their work. Genius, it seemed, was often regarded as a higher calling than personal well-being.

However, the public's attitude was not entirely sympathetic. Critics of Vico's lifestyle saw his physical decline as a failure to live in accordance with the moral and social expectations of the time. In 18th-century Europe, the pursuit of knowledge was still often framed within the context of a balanced life, one where intellectual rigor was expected to coexist with physical vitality. To some, Vico's self-imposed starvation appeared reckless, even irresponsible. His intellectual obsession, they argued, was no excuse for his refusal to maintain basic health practices.

Vico's declining health also raised questions about the mental state of the philosopher. His failure to maintain his health became emblematic of a larger cultural debate on the cost of genius. Was it possible to be an extraordinary thinker and still be a responsible human being? Or did the very nature of genius demand sacrifice—especially of one's own well-being?

How Vico's Health Affected His Work

As Vico's health continued to fail, his ability to write and produce work became increasingly hindered. His physical state, including frequent bouts of weakness, dizziness, and cognitive cloudiness, started to interfere with his intellectual output. It became evident that his work on the *Scienza Nuova* and other philosophical writings had slowed to a crawl. This period of intellectual paralysis was particularly painful for Vico, who had dedicated his life to the development of his ideas.

His late writings, while still filled with brilliant insights, were marked by a noticeable decline in clarity and coherence. The philosopher's handwriting grew more erratic, and his ability to organize his thoughts deteriorated. It was as though the rigor of his intellectual pursuits was draining him of the strength needed to maintain the very mental faculties that had made him famous.

As his physical condition worsened, Vico's social circle became smaller. His friends, once eager to discuss his ideas, found it increasingly difficult to engage with him. Even his most devoted supporters began to turn away, perhaps not out of malice but out of concern for their own health. Vico's mind remained sharp for much of his life, but his body could no longer keep up. The once-formidable philosopher, who had reshaped the way we think about history and culture, was now reduced to a shadow of his former self, his health irreparably damaged by his intellectual obsession.

Public Opinion on Genius and Health

Vico's tragic decline serves as a powerful commentary on the relationship between genius and health in the 18th century. The public, and even his close friends, could not reconcile the brilliance of his mind with the destruction of his body. In a time when intellectualism was still held in high regard, Vico's collapse highlighted the dangers of intellectual isolation and self-neglect.

For some, Vico's obsession with his work seemed almost noble, a testament to the lengths one would go to in the pursuit of knowledge. But for others, his self-imposed suffering was a warning: genius, while precious, was no excuse for neglecting the body's basic needs. The philosopher's untimely death in 1744 at the age of 76, likely hastened by years of self-imposed starvation, left behind not only a brilliant body of work but also a poignant example of the price of intellectual obsession.

Vico's case remains an enduring mystery. His legacy, in both philosophy and history, is indelible, but it is forever intertwined with the tragic cost of his dedication to his ideas—an intellectual life that led to the quiet destruction of the man himself.

8

The Sleep Deprivation of Civil War Soldier Ambrose Bierce

Ambrose Bierce, the American writer and Civil War veteran, is best known for his sharply critical and often chilling depictions of war and death.

His most famous works, including *An Occurrence at Owl Creek Bridge* and *The Devil's Dictionary*, are filled with dark, cynical insights into the nature of humanity, often framed by his personal experiences during the American Civil War. What many do not realize, however, is that Bierce's gloomy worldview and his later writings were deeply shaped by the trauma he endured on the battlefield—not just from the violence he witnessed, but also from the physical and psychological toll of extreme sleep deprivation.

Bierce's time as a soldier, especially his harrowing experiences during the Battle of Shiloh, exposed him to the grim realities of war. Alongside the relentless suffering and death he encountered, Bierce's severe lack of sleep during and after the battles would have far-reaching effects on his mental health, contributing to what we now recognize as post-traumatic stress disorder (PTSD). The long nights spent in constant alertness, the fear of death, and the exhaustion from endless combat would manifest in ways that shaped Bierce's later writing and public persona.

The Soldier's Strain: Sleep Deprivation on the Battlefield

Ambrose Bierce enlisted as a volunteer in the Union Army at the age of 18, eager to serve in a cause he believed in. But the brutal realities of war soon shattered any romanticized notions he had about combat. One of the most taxing aspects of his experience was the severe lack of sleep. Civil War soldiers rarely had the luxury of a proper rest, especially during active combat. Long marches, constant vigilance during night duty, and the fear of being attacked all conspired to leave soldiers like Bierce chronically sleep-deprived.

Bierce's personal account of the Battle of Shiloh, one of the bloodiest engagements of the war, provides a stark picture of the exhausting conditions soldiers faced. In his memoir *What I Saw of Shiloh*, Bierce describes the chaotic and bloody aftermath of the battle, which left 23,000 men dead, wounded, or missing. He recounts the emotional toll the battle took, but also the physical exhaustion: sleepless nights spent on the edge of death, the constant threat of attack, and the inability to properly rest or recover. The noise, the fear, and the stress kept him—and many others—on edge, stripping away their ability to sleep.

Bierce, like countless others in the war, was subjected to the constant state of hyper-vigilance that sleep deprivation induces. This prolonged lack of rest and recovery would have had profound effects on his mind and body, contributing to the psychological toll of the war.

Sleep Deprivation and the Development of PTSD

The modern understanding of post-traumatic stress disorder (PTSD) was not developed until much later, but the symptoms Bierce experienced following his time in the war are now easily recognizable. Chronic insomnia, nightmares, heightened anxiety, and emotional numbness were common effects of sleep deprivation, particularly among soldiers returning from combat. These symptoms are now understood to be part of PTSD, a condition triggered by traumatic experiences that disrupt the mind's ability to process fear and danger.

Bierce's insomnia, fueled by his battlefield experiences, was likely one of the early signs of PTSD. He described vivid and often disturbing dreams, haunted by memories of the war. The mental strain of combat—combined with his sleeplessness—left him in a constant state of emotional turmoil. He became increasingly withdrawn, finding it difficult to connect with the world outside the horrors he had witnessed.

While sleep deprivation itself doesn't directly cause PTSD, it is a significant factor that exacerbates its development. The inability to rest, combined with the constant re-living of traumatic experiences, creates a cycle that intensifies the disorder. Bierce's writing reflects this profound disturbance. His stories often feature protagonists trapped in nightmarish realities, where the line between life and death is blurred, and time itself seems to lose its meaning. These themes resonate strongly with someone who has been deprived of the basic function of sleep for extended periods.

Bierce's Writing: A Reflection of War and Its Effects

Bierce's literary career, in many ways, serves as a testimony to the toll that war took on his mind and body. His work after the war is filled with disillusionment, sharp cynicism, and a dark view of humanity—

traits that can be traced back to his battle experiences and the sleep deprivation that accompanied them. His most famous short story, *An Occurrence at Owl Creek Bridge*, is a haunting tale of a man on the verge of death, struggling to come to terms with his reality. The story's surreal quality—where the passage of time seems suspended and reality distorts—echoes Bierce's own disorientation from his lack of sleep and ongoing trauma.

Another aspect of his writing that reflects his war experiences is his penchant for portraying the futility and absurdity of human endeavor. In his *Devil's Dictionary*, Bierce satirizes human institutions and behaviors with biting humor, revealing his disillusionment with the world around him. This pessimistic worldview can be traced back to his exposure to the horrors of war and the toll it took on his psyche. Sleep deprivation, combined with the overwhelming violence and chaos of the battlefield, left Bierce with a deeply cynical outlook on life, one that pervaded his fiction and nonfiction alike.

In his memoir *What I Saw of Shiloh*, Bierce does not just recount the battle itself; he also reflects on the psychological and emotional toll it took on him. The constant barrage of gunfire, the mass casualties, and the intense fear of death created an environment where rest was not just rare—it was virtually impossible. His inability to sleep during and after the battle left him in a state of heightened sensitivity and paranoia, which is evident in his narrative style.

Public Opinion: The Silent Epidemic of War Trauma

While Bierce's personal experiences with sleep deprivation and PTSD were not well understood in his time, they were certainly not unique. During the Civil War, many soldiers struggled with the aftermath of combat, though the term "shell shock" (later recognized as PTSD) had not yet been coined. The public perception of soldiers' mental health at the time was limited, often overshadowed by the physical injuries they sustained.

There was little recognition that mental trauma could have such profound effects on a person's health. Soldiers returning home were often viewed as "broken" or "unfit," but their struggles with war-induced insomnia, nightmares, and paranoia were dismissed as mere weakness. Some soldiers were even branded as cowards or failures for their inability to adjust to civilian life.

Bierce's writings, however, helped shine a light on the emotional and psychological toll of war. He was not alone in his suffering, but his literary legacy provided a powerful voice for others who were silenced by their trauma. Through his stories, Bierce documented the unseen scars of war—those that could not be treated by medicine or surgery but could only be understood through experience and empathy.

The public's reaction to his work often reflected the same disconnection between society and the psychological wounds of war. Many people were fascinated by his darkly existential tales, but few recognized the personal cost behind them. The emphasis on Bierce's literary genius often overshadowed the depth of his trauma, and his mental health struggles remained hidden behind the veil of his literary success.

Bierce's Legacy: A Voice for the Unseen Wounds of War

Ambrose Bierce's life and work serve as a potent reminder of the mental and physical toll that war takes on those who experience it. His struggles with sleep deprivation and the resulting psychological effects illustrate a broader, often overlooked aspect of warfare: the unseen wounds that last long after the battle is over. His inability to sleep, his vivid nightmares, and his disillusionment with society are all part of a larger narrative of post-war trauma that was largely ignored during his time.

Bierce's stories, which often depict characters trapped in distorted realities, stand as a reflection of his own war-induced disorientation. His work not only provides a chilling portrayal of the Civil War but also offers a window into the psychological costs of combat—a subject that was largely ignored in the public discourse of the time. In examining his insomnia and trauma, we gain a deeper understanding of the complex relationship between war and the human mind, and how sleep deprivation, once thought to be a minor ailment, can have devastating effects on those who endure it.

9

The Breathing Collapse of John Keats

The life of John Keats, the brilliant English Romantic poet, was tragically short, ending at just 25 years old.

Yet, within that brief span, he produced some of the most profound and enduring works in the English language. Keats is celebrated for his lyrical beauty, his vivid exploration of nature, and his deep reflections on love, death, and beauty. However, his legacy as a poet is often overshadowed by the personal suffering he endured due to tuberculosis, the disease that not only robbed him of his physical strength but also shaped much of his emotional and intellectual life.

Keats's battle with tuberculosis (then known as "consumption") was marked by severe respiratory issues that affected his ability to write, think, and even engage with the world around him. As he struggled to breathe, his poems became increasingly tinged with a sense of melancholy and preoccupation with death. In many ways, his short life was defined by his inability to escape the slow and painful collapse of his body, exacerbated by the medical limitations of his time and the poor air quality that accompanied urban life in early 19th-century England.

The Early Signs and the Strain of Tuberculosis

Keats's health problems first became apparent in 1818, when he began suffering from a persistent cough and bouts of fever. It wasn't long before his condition worsened, and by 1820, he was officially diagnosed with tuberculosis. In the years that followed, his physical and emotional well-being would be increasingly dictated by the disease. The constant difficulty breathing became a hallmark of his condition, and Keats found it increasingly difficult to carry out the most basic activities, let alone write.

Tuberculosis primarily affects the lungs, causing a persistent cough, chest pain, fatigue, and, eventually, significant breathing difficulties as the disease progresses. For Keats, the disease not only threatened his life but also restricted his creative output. He was often unable to write for long periods of time due to his worsening health, and his struggle for breath left him feeling weak and drained, both physically and mentally.

In the midst of this battle, Keats's medical options were limited. The disease had no effective treatment at the time, and his doctors could do little more than offer him rest and the standard remedies of the day, none of which could address the root cause of his illness. The impact of tuberculosis on Keats's lungs meant that every breath became a laborious task, and the inability to breathe properly further eroded his energy and spirit.

Keats's Emotional Struggles: Letters to Fanny Brawne

Keats's relationship with Fanny Brawne, his fiancée, is one of the most poignant aspects of his life and work. The two were deeply in love, but their relationship was marred by the progression of Keats's illness. Throughout their correspondence, Keats's letters reveal the deep emotional toll that his physical deterioration had on him. He frequently expressed his frustration at being unable to live the full life he had imagined, particularly with Fanny.

One of Keats's most revealing letters to Fanny is dated 1819, where he writes: *"I have been half in love with you all my life, but I am afraid I am too weak to make any declaration."* These words capture both the longing and resignation that Keats felt in his final years. Despite his love for Fanny, he was fully aware that his time was limited, and his illness rendered any future together uncertain. Keats's inability to breathe freely and his general weakness made even the simplest pleasures, like spending time with Fanny, increasingly difficult.

As his health continued to decline, Keats's letters to Fanny became more desperate, filled with signs of his frustration and despair. He often spoke about his difficulty breathing, the constant coughing fits that left him exhausted, and the emotional toll of knowing that his future was limited. His relationship with Fanny, full of tender moments and painful goodbyes, was overshadowed by his slow decline.

In one particularly poignant letter, Keats writes to Fanny: *"I can't think of you without the dread that I may not live to see you again. The days pass and I can't catch my breath, but I'll try to write some lines if I can still find the strength to do so."* This letter is an encapsulation of the delicate balance Keats had to maintain between his love for Fanny and the physical limitations his body imposed on him. His love for her was undeniable, but it was also intertwined with the cruel reality of his mortality.

Keats's Creative Vision Amidst Physical Collapse

Despite the challenges posed by tuberculosis, Keats produced some of his greatest work during the years when his health was rapidly deteriorating. Works like *Ode to a Nightingale*, *Ode on a Grecian Urn*, and *To Autumn* were written when he was deeply affected by the disease. His art became a way for him to transcend the physical pain he was experiencing, even if only for a fleeting moment.

In *Ode to a Nightingale*, Keats explores the themes of mortality, the fleeting nature of life, and the contrast between human suffering and eternal beauty. This piece reflects his growing awareness of the limitations of his own life and the inevitability of death. The line *"Thou wast not born for death, immortal Bird!"* speaks to the distance Keats felt between the immortality of art and the fragility of his own body.

Similarly, in *Ode on a Grecian Urn*, Keats contemplates the permanence of art and the ephemeral nature of human experience. His work is filled with an awareness of his own physical fragility, yet his creative vision allowed him to reach for something beyond the limits of his failing health.

But even as Keats produced these remarkable poems, his physical suffering was ever-present. His breathing problems made writing more difficult, as the act of creating—an intensely physical process—was often impeded by his compromised health. Tuberculosis robbed him not only of his strength but also of his ability to fully engage with the world, leaving him to channel his remaining energy into writing that would, in the end, immortalize him.

Public Reaction and the Tragic End

Keats's death, on February 23, 1821, was a profound loss for the literary world. At just 25 years old, he was a poet of extraordinary promise, with an entire life of creative potential tragically cut short. His death was mourned by friends, fellow writers, and the public alike. In particular, the romantic notion of the "sick poet" who lived and wrote in the shadow of his own mortality deeply resonated with the public of the time.

In the years following Keats's death, the public continued to mourn what was seen as a life snuffed out too soon. Keats's death became part of the larger myth of the tormented, prematurely-dead genius. His reputation was posthumously elevated, and his works gained greater recognition after his passing. The tragedy of his death, combined with the beauty of his poetry, led to his inclusion among the greatest poets in English literature.

But even as Keats's works were lauded, the circumstances of his death reveal much about the limitations of medicine in the early 19th century. Tuberculosis was a common killer, and the poor air quality in London—coupled with the lack of effective treatments—made the disease all the more lethal. In Keats's case, this combination of environmental and medical factors sealed his fate. His struggle to breathe was not just a physical hardship but also a symbol of the stifling of his genius by forces outside of his control.

Keats's life and death serve as a tragic reminder of the fragility of life, particularly for those living in eras before modern medicine could offer effective treatments. His work, however, endures as a testament to his resilience, his creative genius, and his ability to express the human condition in ways that continue to resonate today.

10

The Stress-Fueled Death of Alexander the Great

Alexander the Great, one of history's most celebrated and enigmatic leaders, died at the tender age of 32.

His early death has remained a subject of fascination and speculation for centuries. While the cause of his sudden illness and death is still debated, it is widely believed that a combination of his intense workload, relentless military campaigns, stress, lack of rest, and possibly heavy drinking played a significant role in his demise. The consequences of Alexander's unsustainable lifestyle, compounded by the tremendous mental and physical strain of ruling an empire that stretched from Greece to India, appear to have ultimately caught up with him.

In the days following his death, ancient sources, such as Plutarch and Arrian, offered various explanations for what killed the Macedonian king. Some suggest that a fever caused by a physical illness, like malaria or typhoid, was the immediate cause, while others argue that the stress of constant warfare and the immense pressures of empire-building may have played a far more significant role. Regardless of the exact medical cause, Alexander's death marked the tragic and premature end of one of the most brilliant military careers in history—one that had reshaped the known world.

The Unrelenting Pace of Conquest

At the time of his death in 323 BCE, Alexander the Great had achieved a level of conquest and empire-building unmatched in history. His military genius, strategic prowess, and unyielding ambition had led him from Greece to Egypt, through Persia, and all the way to India. His armies had fought—and won—dozens of battles, many of which were brutal and long-lasting. The constant movement and preparation for war, combined with the challenges of maintaining control over a vast and diverse empire, left Alexander with little time for rest or recuperation.

From the moment he took the throne at age 20, Alexander's life was defined by war and expansion. Over the next 12 years, he led his army through one campaign after another. In the process, he experienced extreme stress from the demands of leadership and the challenges of commanding an army of tens of thousands. Alexander's commitment to pushing ever forward—often to the point of exhaustion—was legendary, but this very drive would eventually contribute to his physical collapse.

The relentless pace of military campaigns, often accompanied by long marches in extreme climates, would have severely strained Alexander's body. Under these conditions, it would have been nearly impossible to maintain a healthy lifestyle. He was constantly moving from one battlefield to the next, without regular breaks or time to recover from the mental and physical exhaustion that came with such an intense military and leadership role.

The Role of Sleep Deprivation and Stress

One of the more intriguing aspects of Alexander's lifestyle was his notorious lack of rest. Sleep deprivation, particularly chronic sleep deprivation, has been shown to have severe consequences on the human body, both physically and mentally. While the ancient sources do not explicitly mention Alexander's sleep patterns, it is likely that his demanding schedule and the stresses of constant warfare would have left him with little time to sleep or recuperate.

The human body's need for rest is paramount for maintaining immune function and mental clarity. Sleep deprivation weakens the immune system, increases vulnerability to infection, and impairs cognitive function. For someone in Alexander's position—commanding armies, managing vast territories, and dealing with the political complexities of empire-building—the lack of rest would have only compounded the enormous stress he was under.

Stress itself is known to have far-reaching consequences for health. Chronic stress can cause a range of physical problems, including high blood pressure, cardiovascular issues, and a weakened immune system. For Alexander, the pressure of maintaining control over a sprawling empire and the mental strain of leadership would have contributed significantly to his physical decline. As the campaigns wore on, Alexander may have also experienced what we now recognize as burnout: a state of chronic stress that leads to physical and emotional exhaustion.

Heavy Drinking and Its Toll on His Health

Another factor that likely contributed to Alexander's premature death was his heavy drinking, which, according to some ancient accounts, was a regular part of his social and military life. Drinking heavily during feasts, as was common among the Macedonian nobility, may have exacerbated his already weakened physical condition. While it is difficult to know exactly how much alcohol Alexander consumed, reports suggest that he drank to excess, especially in the later years of his campaigns.

Heavy alcohol consumption can be harmful to the body in numerous ways. It weakens the immune system, disrupts sleep patterns, and increases the likelihood of infections. Additionally, alcohol has a dehydrating effect, which, in the context of Alexander's already high-stress lifestyle, may have compounded his physical vulnerabilities.

In the ancient sources, it is noted that in the days leading up to Alexander's illness, he had participated in a particularly heavy drinking session. This is often cited as a factor that may have triggered the onset of the fever that ultimately killed him. Whether or not the drinking directly caused his illness is still a point of debate, but it certainly would have played a role in weakening his health, making him more susceptible to the infections that may have led to his death.

The Fever That Took His Life

By the time Alexander fell ill in the spring of 323 BCE, he had been experiencing the effects of his lifestyle for some time. Ancient historians like Plutarch and Arrian describe the onset of his fever as sudden and severe. According to Plutarch, Alexander developed a fever while at the palace of Nebuchadnezzar II in Babylon. For several days, he suffered from high fever and extreme physical weakness. His condition worsened, and despite efforts by his physicians, he was unable to recover.

The exact nature of the fever that took Alexander's life is still unknown, but modern medical scholars have speculated that he may have contracted a form of malaria, typhoid, or even West Nile virus.

However, considering the stress and exhaustion that Alexander had been enduring, it is also possible that his weakened immune system was unable to fight off a simple infection that would otherwise have been manageable.

The fever lasted several days, and Alexander's strength continued to fade. His inability to rally and his physical deterioration contributed to the sense of despair and inevitability that surrounded his death. According to ancient sources, his last days were filled with agony, and he was unable to fulfill his role as leader and conqueror. The man who had once seemed unstoppable was now helpless, stricken by an illness that his body could not fight.

Public Opinion and the Tragic Loss

At the time of his death, the news spread quickly across the empire, and the reaction was one of shock and disbelief. Alexander the Great was seen as the embodiment of divine strength and leadership. His conquests had brought glory to Greece and Persia, and he was regarded as a hero by many of his subjects. The idea that such a man could die at such a young age, after achieving so much, was a blow to the hopes of his empire.

Public opinion was deeply divided. On one hand, many mourned the loss of a visionary leader, whose death left the empire without a clear successor. On the other hand, some suspected foul play—particularly in the context of Alexander's turbulent relationships with those close to him. Some of his generals and advisors, including his close companion and general Hephaestion, had already died under mysterious circumstances, leading some to believe that Alexander's own death might not have been purely natural.

Despite the speculation, the empire was left in a state of uncertainty. Alexander's sudden and premature death, combined with the rapid deterioration of his health in the months leading up to it, highlighted the toll that stress, lack of rest, and excessive workload can have on the human body—even on one of history's greatest military leaders.

As we reflect on Alexander's death, we see not just the end of a conqueror, but a tragic reminder of the physical and emotional costs of a life led by unrelenting ambition, stress, and the strain of empire-building. The empire Alexander had created did not survive long after his death, splintering into warring factions, further symbolizing the transient nature of even the most extraordinary achievements.

11

The Destructive Obsession of Captain Cook with Perfect Hydration

Captain James Cook, the renowned British explorer, is often celebrated for his groundbreaking voyages to the Pacific, his detailed maps of uncharted territories, and his contributions to the development of navigation and cartography.

Yet, less discussed in the annals of Cook's legacy is his almost obsessive focus on hydration—particularly the prevention of scurvy. While his attention to dietary needs and the health of his crew was undoubtedly groundbreaking at the time, his obsession with the subject, combined with the pressures of leadership during long voyages, ultimately had a profound impact on both his physical health and his relationships with his men.

Cook's efforts to combat scurvy, a disease caused by a lack of vitamin C, played a crucial role in prolonging the lives of sailors during his expeditions, but his singular focus on hydration and nutrition also had unintended consequences. His meticulous measures—though beneficial to some—led to tensions on board, both among the crew and with his superiors. Ironically, despite his innovations and his relentless determination to safeguard the health of his crew, Cook himself was not immune to the effects of poor health, and the stress surrounding his obsessive leadership eventually contributed to his own untimely death.

The Obsession with Hydration and Health

During Cook's era, the physical toll of long voyages was notorious. Sailors faced numerous risks, the most deadly of which was scurvy. Caused by a lack of vitamin C, scurvy led to symptoms such as bleeding gums, fatigue, and ultimately, death. In the mid-18th century, scurvy was a scourge of long-term sea travel. Ships' crews were often plagued by the disease, and there was little understanding of its cause. However, Captain Cook, always the innovative and meticulous leader, was one of the first to propose a solution based on his observations and experiments.

Cook's strategy was simple yet revolutionary for its time: to provide sailors with a regular supply of fresh food, particularly fruits and vegetables, during voyages. This focus on hydration and proper diet was not just an afterthought for Cook—it was a crucial part of his leadership philosophy. As part of his commitment to the health of his crew, Cook enforced strict rules about water quality and vitamin intake. He required that fresh water be collected from the shore whenever possible and ensured that the crew had access to citrus fruits and sauerkraut, which were known to prevent scurvy. His efforts to ensure that his sailors received adequate hydration, proper nutrition, and the right amounts of vitamin C were groundbreaking in an era when most sailors were accustomed to surviving on salted meat and dried biscuits for months on end.

The health of his crew was a constant concern for Cook, and he made sure that his ships were equipped with medical supplies, fresh food, and water purification methods. His journal entries and correspondence often reflect his deep concern for the welfare of his men. He kept detailed records on the provisions used during his voyages, carefully documenting the use of lemon juice and other fresh foods to combat the symptoms of scurvy. His meticulous attention to diet and hydration not only set a new standard for naval health but also contributed significantly to the success of his voyages.

Tensions on Board: The Price of Perfection

Despite Cook's many successes, his obsessive focus on health and hydration came at a cost. His rigorous rules and attention to detail were not always well-received by his crew, many of whom found his strict regulations burdensome. His obsession with perfect hydration and nutrition, though well-intended, led to mounting tensions on board his ships. His men were often subjected to long, monotonous days of work, limited rest, and constant surveillance, all under the watchful eye of their captain.

Cook's leadership style, while effective in many ways, could also be described as authoritarian. He was known to enforce strict discipline on his crew, and his focus on hydration and scurvy prevention became a central aspect of his governance. The constant pressure to comply with these health protocols sometimes led to frustration among sailors, who were not always appreciative of the captain's strict measures. The enforced diet, while essential for their health, was often seen as a burden by those who longed for more freedom or the comfort of traditional rations.

In particular, Cook's obsession with the issue of hydration was problematic when he began to demand that his men drink copious amounts of fresh water, a resource that was often scarce. The constant pursuit of this ideal—combined with the stress of being on long voyages with limited supplies—led to occasional rebellion and discord among his crew members. Some sailors became resentful of Cook's obsessive control over their health, even if it was for their benefit. Tensions surrounding food and hydration on board the ships, combined with the ongoing pressures of exploration, placed an emotional and physical strain on Cook himself, as well as on his leadership.

Cook's Health: The Dangers of Overwork and Stress

Ironically, despite his obsessive care for his crew's health, Captain Cook's own health deteriorated due to the very same pressures he placed on his men. Throughout his voyages, Cook suffered from extreme exhaustion, physical strain, and mental stress, all of which were exacerbated by the demanding conditions of exploration. The stress of leadership—coupled with his intense focus on managing the health of the crew—took a toll on his physical well-being.

Cook's long hours of work, coupled with his tendency to push himself to the limit, led to chronic fatigue. His health gradually worsened during his later voyages, and despite his strict measures to prevent scurvy in his men, Cook himself began to show signs of poor health. His crew members, in their journals, commented on his increasingly frail condition, noting that even the captain himself seemed susceptible to the illnesses that affected his men.

The mental and emotional toll of his obsession with hydration and maintaining strict dietary rules for his crew was also significant. As a leader under constant pressure to maintain discipline and manage every aspect of his crew's health, Cook's mental state began to suffer. His obsessive focus on hydration, while undoubtedly beneficial to the crew in the long term, led to a sense of isolation and stress that likely contributed to his declining health.

The Tragic End: The Cost of Leadership

Despite his commitment to ensuring the survival and well-being of his crew, Captain Cook's life was ultimately cut short. In 1779, on his third and final voyage to the Pacific, Cook was killed in Hawaii during a violent confrontation with the indigenous people. His death was a tragic loss not only for the British Empire but for the entire world of exploration. While his obsession with hydration and nutrition had greatly benefited his crew, it had not been enough to prevent the physical and emotional strain that ultimately led to his demise.

Cook's tragic end was compounded by the public's perception of his leadership and the mixed views on his death. While many mourned the loss of such a brilliant explorer and navigator, others viewed his death as an inevitable consequence of his overwork and obsessive leadership. His insistence on perfect hydration and the strict rules he imposed on his crew may have been seen as symbolic of his inability to balance the demands of leadership with the realities of human frailty. His death, while marking the end of an era of exploration, was also a reminder of the personal toll that obsessive leadership can take, both on the body and on the mind.

In the end, Captain Cook's obsessive focus on hydration and the health of his crew was a double-edged sword. While his innovations in preventing scurvy saved countless lives, the stress and pressures of his relentless pursuit of perfection led to a personal collapse. His life and death serve as a cautionary tale about the dangers of overwork and the toll that obsession can take, even when the intentions behind it are noble and necessary for the survival of others.

12

The Tragic Downfall of the Earl of Essex Due to Sleep Deprivation

```
Robert Devereux, the 2nd Earl of Essex, was once one of the
most admired and promising figures in Elizabethan England.
```

A brilliant military commander and close confidant of Queen Elizabeth I, Essex seemed destined for greatness. His youthful charm, charisma, and military success earned him a prominent place at court. However, by the time of his execution in 1601, Essex had become a symbol of failure and disillusionment. The once-celebrated military leader and court favorite was ultimately brought down by a series of poor decisions, and many historians have pointed to his chronic sleep deprivation as a key factor in his tragic downfall.

Essex's rapid rise to prominence was matched only by his swift and dramatic fall from grace. As a commander, he suffered from a grueling schedule that often deprived him of rest and recovery. His excessive workload, combined with the high-stakes nature of his military campaigns, led to mental and emotional exhaustion that clouded his judgment. The symptoms of sleep deprivation—irritability, poor decision-making, and impaired judgment—played a significant role in his military failures and political missteps. Ultimately, the toll of sleepless nights and increasing stress contributed to his catastrophic defeat in Ireland, his strained relationship with the queen, and his eventual execution for treason.

The Promise of Youth and Early Success

Born in 1566, Robert Devereux was the son of the influential 1st Earl of Essex. His early life promised much, as he was brought up in the royal court and quickly became a favorite of Queen Elizabeth I. By his late teens, Essex had already shown great promise in military matters, and his success during the Spanish Armada campaign in 1588 was seen as a prelude to a brilliant military career.

His relationship with Elizabeth, however, would prove both his greatest asset and his eventual undoing. As a young man, Essex was often compared to the queen's favorite and eventual rival, the Earl of Leicester. His proximity to the monarch made him a central figure in courtly politics, and in the early 1590s, he was granted numerous prestigious titles and appointments, including the position of Lord Lieutenant of Ireland in 1599.

The role in Ireland was a pivotal moment in Essex's life, as it marked the beginning of his decline. The political stakes were high—he was tasked with suppressing the rebellion led by the Catholic forces, who were supported by Spain. This military campaign was seen as essential to maintaining English control over Ireland and securing the crown's authority. However, Essex's leadership during this period would be marred by increasingly erratic behavior, which some contemporaries believed was linked to his growing exhaustion.

The Role of Sleep Deprivation in Military Command

In the months leading up to the failed campaign in Ireland, Essex's mental and physical health began to deteriorate. Military leaders in the 16th century often worked under immense pressure, balancing complex political, strategic, and logistical challenges. The burden of leading a large military force in a foreign and hostile environment, coupled with the constant stress of maintaining a positive relationship with the queen, would have taken a heavy toll on any leader.

For Essex, the symptoms of sleep deprivation were beginning to manifest. The human brain requires rest in order to process complex information, regulate emotions, and maintain cognitive function. Lack of sleep impairs decision-making, memory, and impulse control, which are all essential to military strategy and leadership. Essex's erratic decisions during his Irish campaign—ranging from poorly planned military engagements to an inexplicable decision to retreat from a siege—may have been a direct result of this mental fatigue.

According to contemporary sources, Essex's temper was growing more volatile during this time, and his correspondence with the queen reflected his increasing frustration. In one letter, Essex expressed his concerns about the lack of resources, the loyalty of his men, and the challenges of fighting in a foreign country. Yet, his decisions seemed increasingly detached from reality, as though his ability to think clearly and rationally was eroding under the weight of exhaustion.

Moreover, the Irish campaign was poorly managed due to a series of tactical blunders. Essex's inability to control his forces, his failure to defeat the rebel armies decisively, and his decision to abandon the siege of the rebel stronghold of Kinsale led to widespread disappointment. Essex returned to England in disgrace, and his actions in Ireland were scrutinized as evidence of his failure to effectively lead his troops.

Tensions with the Queen and the Court

When Essex returned to England in the winter of 1599, he was greeted by a queen who was angry and disappointed. Elizabeth had supported his mission to Ireland, and his failure was a direct blow to her authority. Essex's inability to maintain the support of his troops and his erratic behavior—partly attributed to exhaustion—further alienated him from the queen.

During this period, Essex's relationship with Elizabeth began to sour. The queen, in her old age, became increasingly intolerant of failure and disorder. Essex, who had once been the apple of her eye, now found himself out of favor. His rash behavior, including a violent outburst at court, further strained their relationship.

Essex's mental state also deteriorated as he became obsessed with regaining favor at court. He worked tirelessly to repair his standing with Elizabeth, but his efforts were in vain. The stress of trying to salvage his political position, compounded by his exhaustion from the demanding workload, led to a series of miscalculations and failed political maneuvers.

In 1601, Essex found himself involved in the disastrous rebellion known as the "Essex Rebellion." The plot to overthrow Elizabeth and seize control of the government was poorly executed and doomed from the start. Essex's failure to manage his supporters and his impulsive actions—hallmarks of a sleep-deprived, mentally exhausted leader—led to his swift downfall. The rebellion was quickly crushed, and Essex was arrested and charged with treason.

Public Opinion and the Toll of Leadership

Essex's downfall was not only a personal tragedy, but a public spectacle. The English people, who had once seen him as a hero and a symbol of royal ambition, now viewed him as a fallen leader. Some contemporaries were sympathetic to his plight, understanding the immense pressure he faced as a leader in a time of constant warfare and political instability. Others, however, criticized his decisions, blaming his mental instability and poor judgment on his inability to manage the demands of his position.

Many historians and contemporaries have suggested that the stress and exhaustion from years of excessive work led to Essex's tragic fate. His declining health, both physical and mental, is seen as an inevitable consequence of sleep deprivation. As his body failed to recover from the toll of his military campaigns, his mind also began to deteriorate, leading to increasingly poor judgment.

The public's view of Essex was divided, with some seeing his execution as a necessary consequence of his actions, while others mourned the loss of a once-promising leader. His death at the hands of the crown in February 1601 served as a grim reminder of the costs of power and the dangerous effects of prolonged stress, sleep deprivation, and poor decision-making.

Legacy of the Earl of Essex

The life of Robert Devereux, the 2nd Earl of Essex, is a tragic tale of ambition, promise, and ultimate failure. His obsessive drive for success and his inability to manage the pressures of leadership left him vulnerable to mental and physical collapse. Sleep deprivation, combined with the burdens of his military campaigns, contributed significantly to the unraveling of his career and his ultimate death.

Though Essex was a man of remarkable talent and ambition, his inability to balance his work with adequate rest led to his tragic end. His life serves as a poignant reminder of the dangers of relentless pressure and the importance of self-care in maintaining both mental and physical well-being. His downfall remains one of the most fascinating and heartbreaking episodes in the history of Elizabethan England.

13

The Psychological Cost of the 1918 Spanish Flu on Public Leaders

```
The 1918 Spanish flu, one of the deadliest pandemics in human
history, claimed the lives of an estimated 50 million people
worldwide.
```

A s it spread across the globe, it not only wreaked havoc on public health but also placed immense psychological strain on political leaders and public figures who were tasked with managing the crisis. Among them, U.S. President Woodrow Wilson is perhaps the most notable figure whose mental and physical health deteriorated in the face of overwhelming stress and sleep deprivation.

The pandemic, which struck in the midst of World War I, tested the resilience of public leaders as they faced an unprecedented global health crisis. Leaders like Wilson, who were already under enormous pressure due to the demands of war and diplomacy, found themselves grappling with the public's fear, the need for decisive action, and the rapidly rising death toll. Sleep deprivation, stress, and a relentless workload during the Spanish flu not only had physical consequences but also contributed to severe psychological strain that left lasting effects on those at the helm.

The Toll of Leadership During a Crisis

The flu, caused by the H1N1 influenza virus, emerged in early 1918 and spread with alarming speed. Unlike previous flu outbreaks, this strain had an extraordinary mortality rate, and the population was largely unprepared for its ferocity. By the fall of 1918, as the virus reached its peak, the world was already reeling from the devastating impacts of the Great War. Public leaders across the globe were facing immense pressures, trying to lead their nations through both the war and the pandemic.

The United States was no exception. President Woodrow Wilson, already burdened with the complexities of wartime diplomacy and military strategy, found himself thrust into managing a public health disaster of unprecedented scale. With millions of Americans falling ill and death tolls mounting, the pressures on Wilson were immense.

Wilson's leadership during the Spanish flu was marked by a combination of intense stress, lack of sleep, and a heavy workload. At the time, little was understood about the flu virus, and there were no effective treatments. As hospitals overflowed with patients and fear spread through the population, Wilson's role became even more critical. He was expected to provide guidance, instill confidence, and make decisions that would affect the lives of millions.

Yet, despite his prominent position, Wilson was not immune to the physical toll of the flu. As the pandemic swept through Washington, D.C., the president himself became ill in the fall of 1919. However, his illness was not the sole source of his psychological collapse. Long before he contracted the flu, Wilson's mental health was beginning to deteriorate, exacerbated by the exhausting demands of the war and the overwhelming responsibility of managing a global pandemic.

The Case of President Wilson: A Leader's Decline

Woodrow Wilson's health during the final years of his presidency has been the subject of much speculation and analysis. In 1919, shortly after the end of World War I, Wilson embarked on a grueling tour of Europe to promote the League of Nations and the terms of the Treaty of Versailles. His mental and physical health had already begun to show signs of strain, and the intense workload, long hours, and stress only worsened his condition.

Wilson's declining health was not merely the result of the burdens of war and diplomacy; it was compounded by his sleep deprivation, emotional exhaustion, and, as some have speculated, the psychological toll of the Spanish flu. In fact, during his European trip in 1919, Wilson was struck down with a serious illness, possibly a mild stroke or nervous breakdown, that left him incapacitated for several weeks. Historians have suggested that the president's collapse during this period was not simply the result of a single physical illness but the culmination of years of stress and lack of rest.

When Wilson returned to the U.S., his health continued to decline. He had trouble speaking and could no longer manage the daily affairs of the presidency with the same vigor he had before. His condition led to a divided administration, with key advisers—particularly his wife, Edith Wilson—effectively taking on much of his duties. During this time, the public remained largely unaware of the severity of his condition, and much of the responsibility for the post-war negotiations and the pandemic response was left in the hands of his aides.

In retrospect, it is clear that Wilson's exhaustion and the psychological strain from leading a nation through such monumental crises were contributing factors to his decline. The stress of the Spanish flu, combined with the demands of war, fractured Wilson's ability to function. His decision-making became erratic, and his mental faculties seemed to fade, making it difficult for him to effectively address the health crisis or focus on the ongoing demands of his presidency.

The Psychological Burden on Global Leaders

While Wilson is perhaps the most notable example, he was not the only public leader affected by the 1918 Spanish flu. Across the world, political figures who were already under stress due to war or economic challenges found their mental health deteriorating as they struggled to manage the pandemic. The emotional toll on these leaders was immense, as they were forced to make decisions under pressure, while simultaneously trying to protect the health of their people.

In Britain, Prime Minister David Lloyd George was similarly affected. His country, still embroiled in the aftermath of the Great War, was devastated by the flu, which struck at a time when the population was already weakened. Lloyd George's leadership was tested as he grappled with the flu's widespread impact. The public demanded swift and effective action, but the prime minister found himself overwhelmed by the competing crises of war, peace, and the pandemic. The emotional toll on Lloyd George was so great that contemporaries noted his increasingly frail and distracted demeanor.

In France, President Raymond Poincaré also struggled with the stress of leading his country through both the war and the health crisis. The French military, already depleted by the war, was hit hard by the flu. The government faced logistical nightmares as hospitals filled to capacity, and public anxiety soared. Poincaré's response to the flu was marred by the same exhaustion and strain that characterized many world leaders at the time. He too suffered from fatigue and anxiety, and there were even reports of him suffering from physical illnesses that some attributed to the psychological stress he was enduring.

Sleep Deprivation and Its Psychological Toll

The Spanish flu affected millions globally, but the burden on leaders was unique. As heads of state, they were expected to maintain a sense of control and stability, even when they themselves were grappling with fatigue, illness, and a lack of sleep. Sleep deprivation, which is known to impair cognitive function and emotional stability, played a crucial role in the mental collapse of many public figures during the pandemic. For Wilson and others, the relentless demands of leadership and the lack of rest exacerbated their mental exhaustion, making it difficult to respond effectively to the crisis at hand.

Sleep deprivation during the Spanish flu also worsened the psychological toll. Leaders, already working long hours under the stress of global conflict and the health crisis, struggled to sleep. In some cases, their lack of rest resulted in severe mental strain, and their decision-making abilities became increasingly impaired. The inability to rest or recover took a cumulative toll on their physical and emotional well-being, affecting their capacity to lead with clarity and sound judgment.

Public Opinion and the Emotional Impact

The emotional burden on these leaders did not go unnoticed. Newspapers at the time reported on the effects of exhaustion, particularly in the case of President Wilson, whose declining health became a subject of public concern. Journalists and commentators speculated on the mental state of the president, noting his increasing isolation and apparent inability to cope with the demands of the office. While much of the public admired his leadership during the war, his physical and mental decline during the post-war period sparked doubts and fears about his ability to lead through the pandemic.

The emotional toll on leaders also mirrored the experiences of everyday citizens, many of whom were experiencing the same health crisis. In this sense, leaders were not just symbols of political authority—they were also human beings grappling with the same anxiety, fear, and uncertainty as the people they governed.

The Broader Psychological Impact of the Pandemic

The psychological toll of the 1918 Spanish flu was not limited to public leaders. The global scale of the pandemic affected millions, and its emotional and mental health consequences lasted long after the physical symptoms of the disease had subsided. For the leaders who were responsible for managing the crisis, the weight of the pandemic often proved too much to bear, leading to physical breakdowns, mental exhaustion, and a collapse in decision-making.

As history remembers the Spanish flu, it is crucial to recognize the human cost of leadership during such a monumental crisis. While the pandemic exacted an immense toll on the global population, it also left deep psychological scars on the very individuals who were entrusted with guiding their nations through the storm. For figures like Wilson, Lloyd George, and Poincaré, the mental and emotional consequences of the flu were just as devastating as the physical toll. Their experiences stand as a testament to the hidden and often overlooked psychological costs of leadership during times of unparalleled crisis.

14

The Unseen Cost of Living Without Sleep in Ancient Egypt

The awe-inspiring pyramids of Giza have long been a symbol of ancient Egypt's grandeur and architectural genius. However, behind the magnificent stone structures lies a grim reality: the workers who labored to build these colossal monuments were often subjected to grueling conditions, including long hours of work, harsh environmental factors, and little time for rest. While the pyramids themselves remain a marvel of human ingenuity, the cost to those who built them was steep, and one of the most overlooked consequences was the sleep deprivation that likely plagued the workers involved in these monumental projects.

Sleep deprivation in ancient Egypt, though rarely discussed in historical records, can be inferred from various archaeological findings, ancient accounts, and the work schedules imposed on laborers. These men, often farmers and commoners, were pressed into service during the flood season when their agricultural work was halted by the inundation of the Nile River. Their time away from their fields was spent in the quarries and on the construction sites, sometimes enduring extreme conditions for weeks or even months without adequate rest.

The Work Schedule of Ancient Egyptian Laborers

The construction of Egypt's pyramids, particularly the Great Pyramid of Giza, was no small task. Estimates suggest that tens of thousands of workers were involved in the building process, from the quarry workers who cut the stones to the laborers who hauled them into place. Archaeological evidence shows that the workers lived in temporary labor camps near the construction sites, where they were housed and fed in exchange for their labor. However, the demands of their work were intense, and there is no indication that they had sufficient time for sleep, particularly during critical phases of construction.

Egyptian laborers, especially those working on monumental projects, were subject to long hours of physical labor under the harsh sun. The typical workday likely stretched from sunrise to sunset, with only brief breaks for food and water. The intense heat of the Egyptian desert further exacerbated the toll on their bodies, with many workers undoubtedly suffering from dehydration and exhaustion.

The lack of rest, compounded by the exhausting labor, meant that workers were subjected to significant physical and mental strain. Sleep deprivation would have affected not only their physical performance but also their cognitive abilities and overall health. Modern research has shown that sleep is critical for the body's repair processes, immune function, and mental clarity—none of which were accessible to these ancient workers during their extended periods of labor.

Archaeological Evidence of Worker Conditions

Archaeological excavations at the Giza plateau have provided some insight into the lives of the workers who built the pyramids. Excavations of workers' villages, such as the one uncovered at the site of the Great Pyramid, have revealed the harsh realities of their living conditions.

These villages were basic in design, with simple dwellings made of mudbrick. The workers' accommodations were cramped and offered little respite from the intense heat, dust, and noise of the construction site.

Evidence also suggests that the laborers worked in teams, often in rotation, to avoid total exhaustion. However, the long hours they worked likely led to chronic sleep deprivation. With the construction of the pyramids requiring constant labor, it is unlikely that workers were afforded enough time to rest and recover, especially considering the scale of the project. Even if some workers were given brief intervals to recuperate, the psychological and physical toll of their continuous labor would have taken a significant toll on their bodies.

Moreover, studies of skeletal remains found in workers' cemeteries near the pyramids indicate signs of physical stress, such as degenerative joint disease and spinal damage, which are indicative of years of hard labor. These findings suggest that the workers' physical health was compromised by the conditions under which they worked, which would have been further exacerbated by a lack of adequate sleep.

Sleep Deprivation and Its Effects on the Body

The impact of sleep deprivation is well-documented in modern medicine, and it is likely that the ancient Egyptians experienced similar effects. Chronic lack of sleep can lead to a variety of health problems, including weakened immune function, cognitive decline, and increased susceptibility to injury. These symptoms would have been particularly dangerous for the workers, who were performing intense physical labor and operating heavy machinery, such as ramps and levers, to move the massive stones used in the pyramids' construction.

Sleep deprivation also has profound psychological effects. Workers who were deprived of adequate rest would likely have experienced mood swings, irritability, and increased stress, all of which could have diminished their capacity to perform their tasks efficiently. Furthermore, the constant physical strain, combined with insufficient rest, may have led to the development of mental health issues, such as depression or anxiety, which would have gone unrecognized and untreated in ancient times.

Given that sleep is essential for memory consolidation and decision-making, it is likely that the chronic lack of sleep among workers had an impact on their performance. For example, the precision required to cut and transport stones and to construct the complex architectural features of the pyramids would have been compromised by exhaustion. Even slight miscalculations, caused by a lack of sleep or mental fatigue, could have delayed construction timelines or resulted in the waste of valuable resources.

The Societal Context of Sleep Deprivation

In ancient Egypt, the social structure was rigid, and laborers were often at the mercy of the elite, including the pharaoh and his administrators. While the elite class lived in relative comfort, the workers were at the bottom of the social ladder. The work they performed was often seen as a divine duty, especially in the context of pyramid construction, which was believed to be a part of the pharaoh's journey to the afterlife. As such, the work could be both physically and mentally grueling, with little room for individual well-being or self-care.

Sleep deprivation, therefore, was not just a consequence of the work but also a reflection of the broader societal structures that devalued the well-being of workers in favor of large-scale projects designed to glorify the ruling class. The workers had little power to negotiate the conditions under which they worked, and their long hours and inadequate rest were a direct result of a system that prioritized monumental achievement over the health of its people.

This was compounded by the intense environmental conditions in which they worked. The Egyptian climate, with its sweltering heat and arid conditions, made it difficult for workers to stay hydrated and refreshed. The lack of proper hydration, combined with extreme physical exertion and inadequate sleep, would have led to exhaustion and an increased risk of illness. Workers were vulnerable to heatstroke, dehydration, and other illnesses, which would have been further exacerbated by their inability to rest and recover adequately.

The Hidden Cost of Monumental Achievement

The construction of Egypt's pyramids was one of the greatest feats of human labor and engineering in the ancient world. Yet, it came at a hidden cost—the toll it took on the lives and health of the workers who built them. Sleep deprivation, combined with harsh working conditions, likely led to chronic health issues that would have affected their productivity and well-being for years to come. The workers who built these monumental structures did so at great personal sacrifice, often working under conditions that left them exhausted, both physically and mentally.

While the pyramids stand as a testament to ancient Egypt's greatness, they also serve as a reminder of the human cost of monumental achievement. The workers who contributed to their construction are often overlooked in the historical narrative, yet they endured physical and psychological hardships that were rarely acknowledged in their time. In the end, the cost of building these wonders was borne not just by the rulers who commissioned them but by the laborers who worked tirelessly to bring them into existence.

The stories of these workers are lost to time, but the evidence of their sacrifices remains embedded in the stones of the pyramids themselves—

testaments to the grueling work, sleepless nights, and physical tolls that allowed one of the world's greatest civilizations to leave a permanent mark on history.

15

The Final Days of Beethoven: Hydration and Overwork Contributing to Illness

Ludwig van Beethoven, one of the most celebrated and influential composers in Western music history, experienced a gradual and painful physical collapse during the final years of his life. As the composer's fame grew, so did his obsession with perfection in his music, which ultimately led to his demise. His extreme dedication to his craft, combined with neglect for his basic health needs—particularly proper hydration—played a significant role in his physical and mental decline. By the time of his death in 1827, Beethoven was not only struggling with the deafness that had plagued him for much of his life but was also enduring a host of other debilitating health issues, many of which can be attributed to years of overwork, poor habits, and inadequate care.

Beethoven's health issues were not just the result of his deafness but were compounded by his inability to maintain his physical well-being. His obsessive commitment to composing, coupled with his failure to prioritize hydration and rest, contributed significantly to his physical collapse. His final years were marked by excruciating pain, mental exhaustion, and a breakdown of his once-sturdy body. His personal letters, particularly those written to friends and doctors, provide a glimpse into the toll that his extreme work habits and neglect of basic health practices had on his physical and emotional state.

The Strain of Composition and Overwork

Beethoven's relentless pursuit of artistic excellence came at a cost. Known for his obsessive work habits, he would often compose for hours on end, sometimes at the expense of sleep and nutrition. The composer had a well-documented habit of working late into the night, and his passion for his music often meant that he ignored the physical needs of his body. He frequently wrote letters to his friends and doctors about his inability to rest and his dissatisfaction with his health, even as his body began to show signs of deterioration.

In one of his letters to his friend and confidant, the music publisher Franz Wegeler, Beethoven wrote about his exhaustion and physical decline: "I am constantly in pain, yet I cannot stop. I cannot abandon my work. But my body… my body is failing me." His commitment to music was so consuming that he often neglected his hydration, which is believed to have been a significant factor in his deteriorating health.

At the time, the concept of proper hydration was not well understood, and Beethoven's lifestyle only exacerbated his condition. His overwork, compounded by inadequate water intake, likely contributed to chronic dehydration, which would have affected his kidneys, digestive system, and overall energy levels. Dehydration can also cause headaches, fatigue, and muscle cramps—symptoms that Beethoven experienced in his final years.

The Impact of Deafness and Other Physical Ailments

For much of Beethoven's life, he struggled with profound deafness, which began to manifest in his late 20s and worsened as he grew older. The loss of hearing, particularly for someone whose entire existence was centered on music, was a devastating blow. It is believed that Beethoven's frustration with his condition contributed to his mental and physical exhaustion. The deafness caused him significant emotional distress, as he could no longer hear his compositions or engage in musical conversation with others. This, coupled with his growing health problems, left him isolated and withdrawn, consumed by his work.

However, his deafness was not the only ailment that plagued him. Beethoven also suffered from gastrointestinal problems, skin diseases, and severe liver dysfunction in his later years. Historical accounts and medical analysis of Beethoven's remains suggest that he likely suffered from cirrhosis of the liver, possibly due to excessive alcohol consumption. But it was his overwork and poor physical care, including his failure to hydrate properly, that accelerated the decline of his health.

Many contemporary doctors and friends, such as his longtime physician Dr. Johann Peter Frank, expressed concern about Beethoven's condition. Despite their recommendations for rest and moderation, Beethoven stubbornly continued his rigorous work schedule, unwilling to compromise his artistic vision. In a letter to his friend and patron, Archduke Rudolph, Beethoven wrote: "You want me to rest, but how can I rest when I am so consumed by my work? The music does not allow me to be idle." This stubbornness, combined with his disregard for his physical needs, led to an exacerbation of his ailments.

WHEN YOU DON'T SLEEP, DRINK OR BREATHE

The Role of Hydration and Public Reaction

Although Beethoven's personal letters and accounts from his contemporaries do not explicitly link his health problems to dehydration, the signs are suggestive. Chronic dehydration can lead to a variety of health issues, including kidney damage, fatigue, headaches, and impaired cognitive function. Beethoven's deteriorating physical condition—his frequent bouts of illness, fatigue, and stomach pains—suggests that he may have suffered from chronic dehydration. Despite the absence of modern medical understanding, it is clear that Beethoven's neglect of basic hydration played a role in his physical collapse.

In addition to his health issues, Beethoven's increasingly erratic behavior in his final years led to public concern. His intense obsession with composing, coupled with his isolation and emotional turmoil, led some to question his mental state. Letters from his friends and colleagues describe a man who was increasingly irritable and withdrawn, overwhelmed by the demands of his music and the physical limitations imposed by his declining health.

The public's reaction to Beethoven's health problems ranged from sympathy to disbelief. Some saw him as a tragic figure, a man whose genius was marred by his inability to care for his body. Others, particularly in the aristocracy, viewed his declining health with skepticism, attributing his eccentricities to personal flaws rather than the toll of a grueling lifestyle. Beethoven's condition was widely misunderstood at the time, as the effects of chronic overwork and dehydration were not fully understood.

The composer's deafness, combined with his failure to take care of his body, led to a deep sense of frustration. He was haunted by the idea that his best work was behind him, and as he grew weaker, he became consumed by his desire to leave a lasting legacy. Letters to his friends show his increasing despair over his inability to work at the pace he once did: "I am not the man I was. The music comes to me less easily. I feel as though my body is betraying me."

The Physical Collapse of a Genius

By 1827, Beethoven's health had deteriorated to the point that he was no longer able to compose. His body had become frail, and his mind was clouded by pain and exhaustion. His once-vibrant passion for music was overshadowed by the physical and mental toll of his neglect. Despite his failing health, Beethoven's genius remained undiminished, and he continued to create some of his most profound works during his final years, including the Ninth Symphony and the late string quartets.

Beethoven's final days were marked by increasing physical collapse. He had suffered from bouts of extreme exhaustion, digestive problems, and swelling in his legs. His liver had likely become severely compromised due to years of overwork, poor hydration, and possible alcohol consumption. Historical accounts suggest that Beethoven died in his home in Vienna on March 26, 1827, after a prolonged illness.

The cause of Beethoven's death remains a subject of speculation. Some historians believe that he succumbed to complications from cirrhosis of the liver, while others point to the cumulative effects of his years of neglecting his health. What is clear, however, is that Beethoven's health was deeply affected by his obsessive work habits and his inability to maintain a balance between his creative passion and his physical well-being.

A Legacy of Genius and Suffering

Beethoven's life is a testament to the cost of artistic genius and the toll it can take on the human body. While his music continues to inspire and move audiences around the world, the personal sacrifices he made in pursuit of perfection are undeniable. His final years, marked by deafness, physical decline, and emotional suffering, reflect the destructive nature of neglecting one's health in the pursuit of greatness. Beethoven's story serves as a stark reminder of the importance of self-care, and the dangers of allowing one's obsession with work to override basic needs like hydration, rest, and physical maintenance.

Beethoven's legacy, both in music and in the lessons learned from his life, remains profound. His ability to create such powerful music despite his many health struggles is a testament to his indomitable spirit. Yet, his decline also reveals the tragic consequences of living without balance—of pushing oneself beyond human limits and ignoring the fundamental needs of the body.

www.ingramcontent.com/pod-product-compliance
Lightning Source LLC
LaVergne TN
LVHW020607181224
799403LV00025B/435